Placental Pathology

Editor

REBECCA N. BAERGEN

SURGICAL PATHOLOGY CLINICS

surgpath.theclinics.com

Consulting Editor
JOHN R. GOLDBLUM

March 2013 • Volume 6 • Number 1

ELSEVIER

1600 John F. Kennedy Boulevard • Suite 1800 • Philadelphia, Pennsylvania, 19103-2899

http://www.theclinics.com

SURGICAL PATHOLOGY CLINICS Volume 6, Number 1
March 2013 ISSN 1875-9181, ISBN-13: 978-1-4557-7337-4

Editor: Joanne Husovski

Surgical Pathology Clinics (ISSN 1875-9181) is published quarterly by Elsevier Inc., 360 Park Avenue South, New York, NY 10010. Months of issue are March, June, September, and December. Business and Editorial Office: Elsevier Inc., 1600 John F. Kennedy Blvd., Ste. 1800, Philadelphia, PA 19103-2899. Accounting and Circulation Offices: Elsevier Inc., 3251 Riverport Lane, Maryland Heights, MO 63043. Periodicals postage paid at New York, NY and at additional mailing offices. Subscription prices are $191.00 per year (US individuals), $220.00 per year (US institutions), $94.00 per year (US students/residents), $239.00 per year (Canadian individuals), $249.00 per year (Canadian Institutions), $239.00 per year (foreign individuals), $249.00 per year (foreign institutions), and $116.00 per year (international & Canadian students/residents). Foreign air speed delivery is included in all *Clinics'* subscription prices. All prices are subject to change without notice. **POSTMASTER:** Send address changes to *Surgical Pathology Clinics*, Elsevier, 3251 Riverport Lane, Maryland Heights, MO 63043. Customer Service: 1-800-654-2452 (US). From outside the United States, call 1-314-447-8871. Fax: 1-314-447-8029. E-mail: JournalsCustomerServiceusa@elsevier.com (for print support) and JournalsOnlineSupport-usa@elsevier.com (for online support).

Reprints. For copies of 100 or more, of articles in this publication, please contact the Commercial Reprints Department, Elsevier Inc., 360 Park Avenue South, New York, NY 10010-1710. Tel. (212) 633-3812; Fax: (212) 462-1935; E-mail: reprints@elsevier.com.

Contributors

CONSULTING EDITOR

JOHN R. GOLDBLUM, MD
Chairman, Professor of Pathology, Department
of Anatomic Pathology, Cleveland Clinics
Lerner College of Medicine, Cleveland Clinic,
Cleveland, Ohio

EDITOR

REBECCA N. BAERGEN, MD
Professor of Pathology and Laboratory
Medicine, Chief of Perinatal and Obstetric
Pathology, Department of Pathology and
Laboratory Medicine, Weill Medical College
of Cornell University, New York-Presbyterian
Hospital, Weill-Cornell Medical Center,
New York, New York

AUTHORS

REBECCA N. BAERGEN, MD
Professor of Pathology and Laboratory
Medicine, Chief of Perinatal and Obstetric
Pathology, Department of Pathology and
Laboratory Medicine, Weill Medical College of
Cornell University, New York Presbyterian
Hospital, Weill-Cornell Medical Center,
New York, New York

KURT BENIRSCHKE, MD
Professor of Pathology, Emeritus, UCSD
Medical Center, University of California
San Diego, San Diego, California

JOANNA S.Y. CHAN, MD
Assistant Professor, Department of Pathology,
Anatomy, and Cell Biology, Thomas Jefferson
University Hospital, Philadelphia, Pennsylvania

MONIQUE E. DE PAEPE, MD
Staff Pathologist, Department of Pathology,
Women and Infants Hospital; Professor,
Department of Pathology and Laboratory
Medicine, Alpert Medical School of Brown
University, Providence, Rhode Island

LINDA M. ERNST, MD
Assistant Professor of Pathology,
Northwestern University Feinberg School of
Medicine, Chicago, Illinois

ONA MARIE FAYE-PETERSEN, MD
Professor of Pathology and Obstetrics and
Gynecology, The University of Alabama at
Birmingham, Birmingham, Alabama

FÜSUN GÜNDOĞAN, MD
Staff Pathologist, Department of Pathology,
Women and Infants Hospital; Associate
Professor, Department of Pathology and
Laboratory Medicine, Alpert Medical School of
Brown University, Providence, Rhode Island

DEBRA S. HELLER, MD
Professor of Pathology & Laboratory
Medicine, Professor of Obstetrics,
Gynecology, & Women's Health, Department
of Pathology & Laboratory Medicine,
UMDNJ-New Jersey Medical School,
Newark, New Jersey

CYNTHIA KAPLAN, MD
Professor of Pathology, Pathology
Laboratories, State University of New York
Stony Brook, Stony Brook, New York

RAJ P. KAPUR, MD, PhD
Professor of Pathology, Department of
Laboratories, The University of Washington,
Seattle Children's Hospital & Regional Medical
Center, Seattle, Washington

FREDERICK T. KRAUS, MD
Adjunct Professor, Department of
Obstetrics and Gynecology, Washington
University School of Medicine, St Louis,
Missouri

RAYMOND W. REDLINE, MD
Professor of Pathology and Reproductive
Biology, Department of Pathology, Case
Western Reserve University School of
Medicine, University Hospitals Case Medical
Center, Cleveland, Ohio

Contents

Preface: Placental and Perinatal Pathology   ix

Rebecca N. Baergen

Gross Examination of the Placenta   1

Cynthia Kaplan

Gross examination of the placenta is important to identify lesions and prepare material for histologic sectioning. The umbilical cord shows many variations, some of which may be associated with significant perinatal morbidity and mortality. Membranous processes often relate to ascending infection, passage of meconium, or hemorrhage. Many villous lesions are the result of processes in the maternal or fetal circulation. Infarcts are common but need to be carefully identified on gross. Although certain routine histologic sections should be done on all placentas, the gross examination guides the selection and reveals other important aspects of the placenta to evaluate.

Monozygotic Twinning   27

Kurt Benirschke

This article discusses pathologies found in monozygotic twinning. Detailed information is provided regarding the development during monozygotic twin formation: embryo development, twin-to-twin transfusion syndrome, acardiac twinning, vanishing twins, conjoined twins, and Beckwith-Weidmann syndrome twins. An algorithm describing the approach for identifying pathology in a placenta with multiple pregnancies is presented.

Ascending Infection: Acute Chorioamnionitis   33

Füsun Gündoğan and Monique E. De Paepe

Acute chorioamnionitis is a major cause of spontaneous preterm birth, accounting for more than 40% of deliveries complicated by preterm premature rupture of membranes or preterm labor. In the majority of cases, especially in preterm births, acute chorioamnionitis is caused by ascending polymicrobial infection. Recent evidence suggests that in some cases acute chorioamnionitis may have a noninfectious cause. In addition to the nonspecific patterns of conventional acute chorioamnionitis, this article describes characteristic inflammatory patterns indicative of a specific infectious cause. Several inflammatory entities of putative immunologic (noninfectious) etiology are addressed, including eosinophilic/T-cell vasculitis and chronic chorioamnionitis.

Umbilical Cord Pathology   61

Rebecca N. Baergen

Problems and abnormalities of the umbilical cord play a significant role in perinatal morbidity and mortality. Because the umbilical cord is the lifeline of the fetus, any disruption of blood flow through the umbilical vessels can lead to severe fetal consequences.

Fetal Thrombotic Vasculopathy: Perinatal Stroke, Growth Restriction, and Other Sequelae   87

Frederick T. Kraus

Clots in the fetal circulation of the placenta may occlude or narrow the lumens of fetal vessels sufficiently to diminish the placental oxygen and nutritional exchange, causing significant reduction in placental function. When extensive, growth restriction, neonatal encephalopathy, and stillbirth may occur. Propagation of clots in other organs, such as brain, kidney, and liver, may affect the function of these organs, resulting in infarcts and neonatal stroke. This article presents an account of the placenal pathology and clinical sequelae of this condition, called fetal thrombotic vasculopathy.

Maternal Floor Infarction and Massive Perivillous Fibrin Deposition   101

Ona Marie Faye-Petersen and Linda M. Ernst

Maternal floor infarction (MFI) and massive perivillous fibrin deposition (MPVFD) are pathologically overlapping placental disorders with characteristic gross and shared light microscopic features of excessive perivillous deposition of fibrinoid material. Although rare, they are associated with high rates of fetal growth restriction, perinatal morbidity and mortality, and risks of recurrence with fetal death. The cause of the extensive fibrinoid deposition is unknown, but evidence supports involvement of maternal alloimmune or autoimmune mechanisms. This article presents an updated discussion of features, placental histopathologic differential diagnosis, possible causes, clinical correlates, and adverse outcomes of the MFI/MPVFD spectrum.

Villitis of Unknown Etiology and Massive Chronic Intervillositis   115

Joanna S.Y. Chan

Villitis of unknown etiology (VUE) is a common lesion affecting from 6.6% to 33.8% of third-trimester placentas. VUE needs to be distinguished from villitis of infectious etiology, most commonly cytomegalovirus and syphilis. Clinically, this lesion is associated with intrauterine growth retardation, intrauterine fetal demise, fetal neural impairment, maternal alloimmune and autoimmune disease, and maternal hypertension. It has a tendency to recur in subsequent pregnancies. Massive chronic intervillositis, also known as chronic histiocytic intervillositis, is a rare lesion that has an unclear relationship with VUE, which is associated with recurrent abortions.

Placental Mesenchymal Dysplasia   127

Ona Marie Faye-Petersen and Raj P. Kapur

Placental mesenchymal dysplasia is a rare, incompletely understood placental stromal lesion, characterized by placentomegaly and striking ectasia and tortuosity of chorionic plate and stem villous vessels. Its prenatal ultrasonographic and gross pathologic features resemble those of a partial mole, but the fetus is often structurally normal and the placenta has a diploid, chromosomal complement. We discuss the pathologic features and current understanding of the etiopathogenesis of this condition, the supportive immunohistochemical and confirmatory molecular genetic studies important in its diagnosis, and its implications for pregnancy and infant outcomes.

Correlation of Placental Pathology with Perinatal Brain Injury   153

Raymond W. Redline

The purpose of placental pathology is to explain adverse clinical outcomes. One of the most tragic of these outcomes is perinatal brain injury with subsequent neurodisability. Findings in the placenta can play an important role in documenting sentinel events, uncovering clinically silent thromboinflammatory disease processes, revealing developmental alterations in functional reserve, and suggesting alterations in related maternal and fetal physiology. These findings, when integrated with clinical data, provide a plausible explanation for an otherwise unexpected outcome and can be helpful for treating physicians and family members.

Placenta Accreta and Percreta   181

Debra S. Heller

The incidence of abnormally adherent placenta (accreta/percreta) has increased 10-fold in the past 50 years, predominantly due to the increased use of cesarean section delivery. The causes, clinical correlates, and pathology of these conditions are discussed in this article.

Index   199

SURGICAL PATHOLOGY CLINICS

FORTHCOMING ISSUES

Current Concepts in Liver Pathology
Sanjay Kakar, and Dhanpat Jain, *Editors*

Current Concepts in GI Pathology
Jason L. Hornick, *Editor*

Cytopathology
Tarik El Sheikh, *Editor*

RECENT ISSUES

Current Concepts in Molecular Oncology
Jennifer Hunt, MD, *Editor*

Breast Pathology: Diagnosis and Insights
Stuart J. Schnitt, MD, and Sandra J. Shin, MD, *Editors*

Current Concepts in Cardiovascular Pathology
Gayle L. Winters, MD, *Editor*

Preface
Placental and Perinatal Pathology

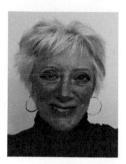

Rebecca N. Baergen, MD
Editor

Placental and perinatal pathology has evolved significantly in recent years. For many pathologists, examination of the placenta has been challenging for several reasons. It is an organ comprising tissue from two individuals and is ever-changing as it matures throughout gestation. It has only been in the last 50 years or so that interest has been sparked in this important organ. Much of this interest is due to the extensive work of Kurt Benirschke and others like him who took on an organ that was often discarded and found that it provided a wealth of information on both the fetus and the mother. There has also been renewed interest from the legal profession as the placenta has taken a major role in adjudicating malpractice cases in obstetrics.

Therefore, it is timely to present a text with practical coverage of the current concepts, diagnostic criteria, differential diagnoses, and pitfalls in the diagnosis of placental lesions. In this volume, we have attempted to bring together a group of the most knowledgeable pathologists in this area to cover a number of important topics in this field.

It has been my honor to have edited this volume and to work with pathologists who are experts in the field. I am deeply indebted to all the authors who contributed to this issue as their knowledge, experience, and expertise in this challenging area of pathology have been invaluable. I would also like to acknowledge Joanne Husovski for her assistance and support in the preparation of this issue. I am also indebted to all my colleagues, fellows, trainees, and, particularly, my mentor, Kurt Benirschke.

Rebecca N. Baergen, MD
Professor of Pathology and Laboratory Medicine
Chief of Perinatal and Obstetric Pathology
New York-Presbyterian Hospital
Weill-Cornell Medical Center
520 East 70th Street, Starr 1002
New York, NY 10065, USA

E-mail address:
rbaergen@med.cornell.edu

Gross Examination of the Placenta

Cynthia Kaplan, MD

KEYWORDS

• Placenta • Gross examination • Umbilical cord • Vascular placental lesions • Placental infection

ABSTRACT

Gross examination of the placenta is important to identify lesions and prepare material for histologic sectioning. The umbilical cord shows many variations, some of which may be associated with significant perinatal morbidity and mortality. Membranous processes often relate to ascending infection, passage of meconium, or hemorrhage. Many villous lesions are the result of processes in the maternal or fetal circulation. Infarcts are common but need to be carefully identified on gross examination. Although certain routine histologic sections should be done on all placentas, the gross examination guides the selection and reveals other important aspects of the placenta to evaluate.

OVERVIEW

A competent gross examination is the important first step in handling surgical pathology specimens; this is especially true for the placenta. Many placental lesions are diagnosed solely by gross examination, and the extent of pathologic processes is best recognized on the whole specimen. The gross examination also guides the choice and number of histologic sections. Ideally, clinical information is available at the time of gross examination, including length of gestation, fetal weight, and any problems related to the pregnancy, birth, or fetus/neonate. Indication for submission is important, because there are many normal variations in placental morphology that may not be appreciated by delivering personnel.

Gross examination of placentas should be done in a systematic routine, so all features are assessed. Special circumstances or lesions may require deviation from this routine. Examination entails specific observations on the cord, peripheral membranes, and fetal and maternal surfaces. The placenta is trimmed of cord, membranes, and excess clot before weighing (**Fig. 1**A), and a roll is created from the membranes to evaluate a large amount of the surface (see **Fig. 1**B). The roll should be made in a manner that includes the point of membrane rupture. Some examiners use a wedge of marginal placental tissue as the core. After inspection of both surfaces, multiple parallel cuts are made from maternal to fetal surface, inspecting and palpating for villous lesions. The basic steps are summarized in the Key Points. The gross placental examination is not a difficult procedure and can be performed rapidly, with experience.[1,2] Photographs of placental abnormalities may be useful for later correlation with microscopic features and clinical aspects. The choice of material for histologic sections needs to be based on gross features, both normal and abnormal. Placentas are heterogenous and overall evaluation can be significantly distorted by suboptimal sectioning.

Examination of placentas can occur in either the fresh or fixed state. Primary formalin fixation makes placentas less infectious and easier to section but eliminates the possibility of fresh tissue for karyotype or DNA procurement. Complete fixation of a whole placenta takes many days in adequate amounts of formalin, something not usually possible in a hospital setting. There are also increasing concerns related to formalin exposure for pathology personnel, and gross examination of previously fixed placentas requires an appropriate area.[3] Fresh examination with fixation of samples for histologic sectioning eliminates considerable formalin exposure and allows special studies. The remainder of the placenta may be

The author has nothing to disclose.

Pathology Laboratories, University Hospital Level II, State University of New York Stony Brook, Stony Brook, NY 11794-7025, USA

E-mail address: Cynthia.kaplan@sbumed.org

Surgical Pathology 6 (2013) 1–26

http://dx.doi.org/10.1016/j.path.2012.11.001

surgpath.theclinics.com

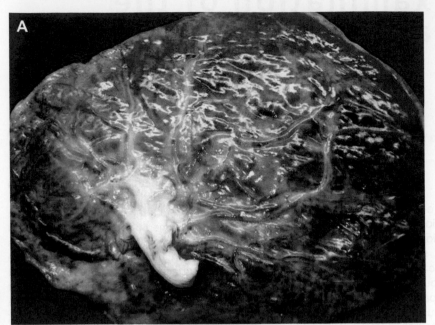

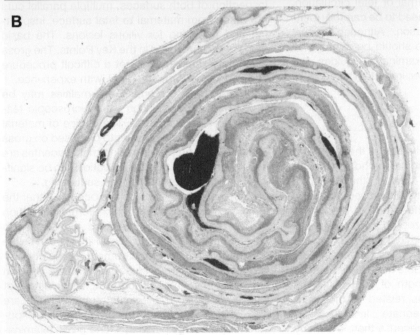

Fig. 1. (*A*) Fetal surface of a trimmed term placenta shows a moderate amount of subchorionic fibrin deposition. The umbilical cord is inserted eccentrically, close to the margin. The majority of the branch vessels of the cord traverse in one direction. (*B*) Scan of section of membrane roll. There is amnion, chorion, and attached decidua, which may contain maternal vessels (hematoxylin and eosin ×2).

Stored in formalin or discarded in most cases. Bouin fixative can also be used with the appropriate procedures for processes. Some examiners prefer this because it hardens the placental tissue and makes it easier to cut blocks. New fixatives without formalin have been formulated to lessen exposure. Unfortunately, they are not useful for the placenta because they do not adequately preserve the tissue and create a variety of artifacts on gross and microscopic.

Although it is possible to cut blocks from fresh placental tissue, it is easier after some fixation has occurred. On most placentas, cord cross-sections (2 pieces from different sites), membrane roll, and 2 to 3 full-thickness pieces of villous tissue, including fetal and maternal surfaces, are an adequate sample. The pieces of placental villous tissue should be from separate areas (different cotyledons) and not from the margin of the placenta, which frequently shows changes of diminished blood flow and fibrin deposition. The fetal surface of the villous section should include small blood vessels and be free of substantial subchorionic clot or fibrin. Early changes of ascending infection are often masked in areas with thick subchorionic deposits. The amnion detaches readily from the chorion and can be easily lost. Additional blocks with representative sections of significant lesions or differences in villous character are also taken. It is not necessary to section every infarct, hemorrhagic lesion, and so forth, as long as they are clearly identifiable grossly and are adequately described.

GROSS LESIONS OF THE PLACENTA

PLACENTAL WEIGHT

Placental weight can vary considerably because it is affected by fixation, the presence of cord, membranes, and loose clot, the amount of blood retained, and the intactness of the maternal surface. Fresh refrigerated placentas lose a small amount of weight with storage, whereas formalin fixation leads to an increase, no more than 5% in either case.[4] Knowing the gestational age and weight of the baby are important to appropriately evaluate the measured weight, and the fetal/placental weight ratio can be readily calculated during the grossing process. The ratio increases from approximately 2 at 20 weeks to approximately 7 to 8 at term.[5,6] A heavy or light placenta often indicates an abnormal pregnancy. Term placentas generally weigh between 400 g and 600 g. There are standard tables for placental weight by gestational age and by fetal weight available.[7–9]

SHAPE

Although the placenta shows extensive growth and histologic change in the second and third trimesters, the basic gross morphology is established early in pregnancy, before the end of the first trimester. The shape of the placenta is variable. Generally it is round to ovoid and approximately 18-cm to 20-cm diameter by 1.5-cm to 2.5-cm thick at term (see **Fig. 1**B). Failure of atrophy of capsular villi leads to succenturiate lobes (**Fig. 2**). Bilobate placentas result from lateral uterine sulcal implantation whereas unusually shaped or multilobate placentas may be due to uterine cavity abnormalities. These alterations should be generally and/or briefly described. Such unusual shapes may have problems related to compression or rupture of the membranous (velamentous) vessels that often accompany them. There is also literature suggesting the

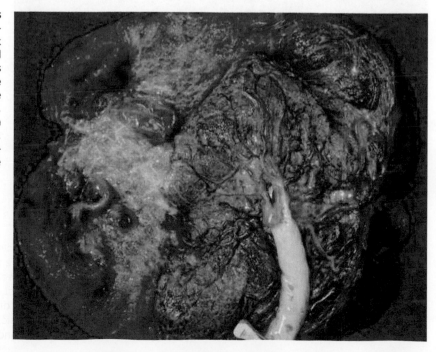

Fig. 2. This placenta is from a patient with placenta previa. Several dark brown masses are noted in the membranes of this placenta away from the main placental disc. These are succenturiate lobes, extra portions of placenta that failed to atrophy. Velamentous vessels typically connect these to the main placental disc.

amount of villous tissue necessary for fetal growth may in part depend on the shape and thickness of the placenta.[10,11]

When implantation occurs low in the uterus, in a vaginal delivery, the point of membrane rupture is near the placental edge. True placenta previa occurs when placental villous tissue covers the cervical opening. This process is often difficult to confirm on placental examination, particularly if there has not been significant clinical bleeding. The maternal surface may show old or fresh hemorrhage or merely a 1-cm to 2-cm circular deposition of fibrin in the region of the cervix. In the setting of placenta previa, other complications frequently occur. Premature separation of the placenta in the region of the cervical os is associated with bleeding. There is often poorly developed decidua or scarring in the lower uterine segment, the site of implantation in placenta previa. This predisposes to placenta accreta and other forms of abnormally adherent placentas.

UMBILICAL CORD

The umbilical cord is the lifeline of the fetus. Complete cord occlusion quickly leads to fetal demise whereas intermittent obstruction has been associated with intrauterine brain damage.

Intrinsic and extrinsic cord compressions are important factors in fetal distress. Careful gross umbilical cord examination often reveals significant lesions that may be associated with cord compromise.

The umbilical cord forms in the region of the body stalk where the embryo is attached to the chorion. This area contains the allantois, omphalomesenteric duct, vitelline vessels, and evolving umbilical vessels. The expanding amnion surrounds these structures and covers the umbilical cord. Eventually, most of the embryonic elements and the right umbilical vein disappear, leaving 2 arteries and 1 vein. Embryologic remnants are rarely visible grossly.

The absence of one umbilical artery is a common anomaly, occurring in approximately 1% of deliveries (**Fig. 3**). It is more frequent with multiple gestation and velamentous cord insertions. Approximately 20% of infants missing one artery have other major congenital anomalies, which may involve any organ system. Several cuts along the cord length should confirm this finding because the two umbilical arteries frequently fuse just above the insertion site.

The spiral twisting of the cord is established early in development. Most commonly it is counterclockwise, a so-called left twist (**Fig. 4**). The

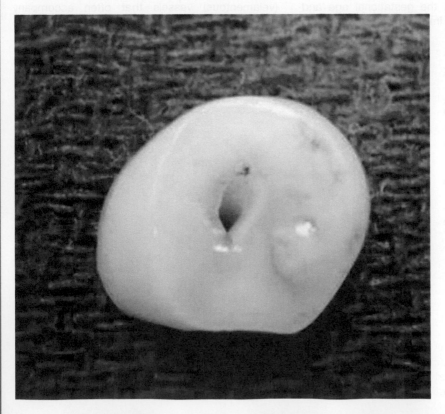

Fig. 3. Cross-section of umbilical cord with single umbilical artery. The vein tends to be larger than the arteries in most cords.

Fig. 4. The vast majority of umbilical cords twist in a counterclockwise manner or left twist, which appears as the left side of the letter "V". Cords may also have little or no twist or twist clockwise (right side of the letter "V"). The cord generally twists every 2 cm to 3 cm of length. Cords with significantly higher numbers of twists and possibly those without twist have higher associated morbidity and mortality. The cord with the left twist shows a false knot, a redundancy of the vein. These can be large but have never been associated with problems.

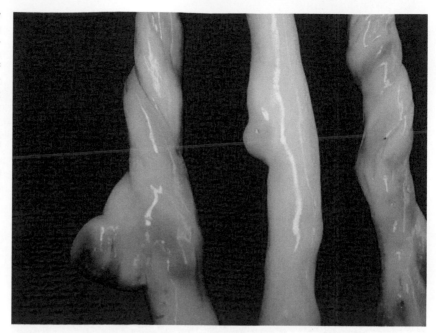

cause of twisting is unknown but seems to create more functional blood flow and helps protect the vein from compression. The number of twists in the cord can be counted and excessive twisting is associated with fetal morbidity and mortality.[12] In general, caution should be used in attributing fetal death to cord problems, particularly if congestion and/or thrombosis is absent. It may one of several contributing factors or truly incidental.

One of the most obvious features of the umbilical cord is the length, which increases throughout gestation, although the growth rate slows in the third trimester. Fetal activity and stretch on the cord are major factors determining length and there is a genetic component. Both abnormally long and short cords have significant clinical correlates. Long cords (greater than 75 cm) are well associated with knots and fetal entanglements (**Fig. 5**). Congestion and thrombosis in cord vessels are helpful signs of true obstruction. A minimum cord length of 32 cm is believed necessary for normal vaginal delivery. Undue traction on a short cord can cause fetal distress, cord tearing with hemorrhage, and possibly placental separation. Fortunately, this is rare. The majority of hemorrhages in the cord are associated with clamp marks are artifacts (**Fig. 6**). Entanglement can lead to a functionally short cord. Short

cords are known to occur in disorders with decreased fetal movement and statistically show more problems in neurologic development. Although it is important to measure the entire cord length received, a true measure is ideally done at delivery.

Premature infants tend to have thicker umbilical cords than more mature babies, whereas cord substance is often lacking and cords are thin in uteroplacental insufficiency. Edema of the cord can be impressive (see **Fig. 6**) but, outside of hydrops, has no known clinical significance. Cord diameter varies considerably along the length and is generally thicker near the infant. Isolated areas of true cord stricture occur, particularly near the fetal body wall and at the placenta to cord insertion (**Fig. 7**).

The insertion of the cord is normally into the placental disc in a central or near central location (see **Fig. 1**). Much eccentricity may be related to unequal placental growth later in pregnancy, generally toward the fundus. Velamentous vessels are particularly important to evaluate and document, because they are associated with compression or rupture (**Fig. 8**). Although usually seen with velamentous insertions, small membranous vessels can be present along the edge with normal insertions. The vessels in the cord may separate

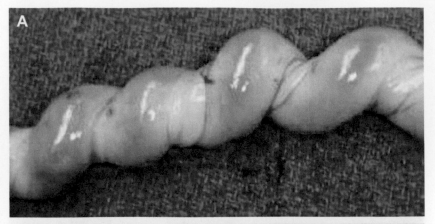

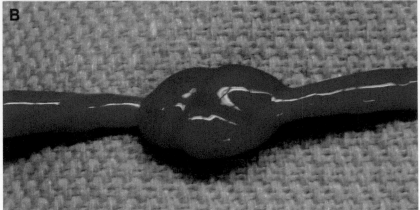

Fig. 5. (*A*) This cord had more than the usual number of twists along its entire length. The vein is dilated and can be seen through Wharton jelly. (*B*) Complicated true knot in an abnormally long umbilical cord. This was a preterm pregnancy with an intrauterine demise. Cord accidents occur at all gestational ages.

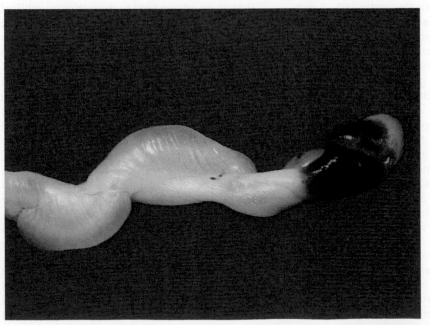

Fig. 6. The cord diameter here is increased by the accumulation of fluid in Wharton jelly. Severe edema may be extreme, widening the cord to several centimeters diameter. Even in severe cases, there is no recognized associated pathology. Near the 3-o'clock position, there is a delivery clamp mark associated with hemorrhage. Most hemorrhages within the cord are artifact and sections should be taken from other areas.

Fig. 7. The true stricture within the midportion of the umbilical cord led to fetal demise. Strictures and torsion are more common near the fetal and placental cord insertions and are not postmortem artifacts.

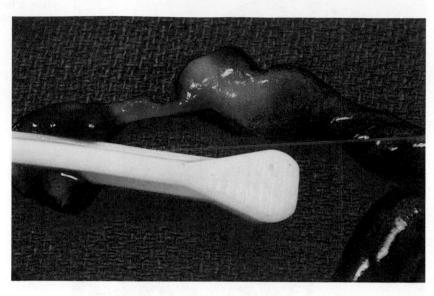

before it reaches the surface (furcate) (**Fig. 9**). The surface amnion may also attach to the cord as a web several centimeters before the cord reaches the placental surface (**Fig. 10**).

The cord inflammation seen with common ascending infections is usually not recognizable grossly. Candida is an exception and shows characteristic microabscesses on the cord surface (**Fig. 11**). Chronic necrotizing funisitis shows perivascular calcification and likely represents a chronic and sometimes healed intrauterine infection with organisms of low virulence (**Fig. 12**). At times, the cord has a yellow color with significant cord inflammation or is stained green with meconium exposure (**Fig. 13**).

Longstanding exposure to bile or meconium may lead to a loss of Wharton jelly with ulceration of the cord. Complete thrombosis of one umbilical

Fig. 8. In this velamentous insertion of the cord, the cord enters the membranes and branch vessels traverse the distance to the placental disc and can be ruptured or compressed. The length of the velamentous vessels is variable. They are short in this example.

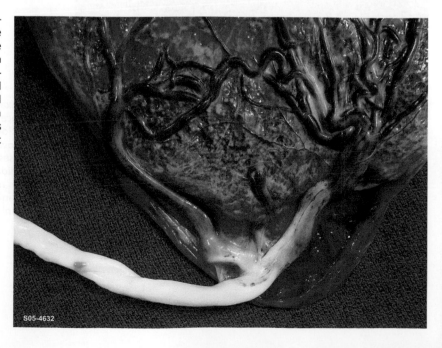

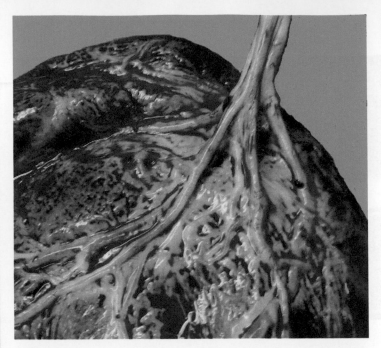

Fig. 9. The umbilical cord divides into branch vessels above the chorionic plate, a furcate insertion. These have similar risks to other velamentous vessels.

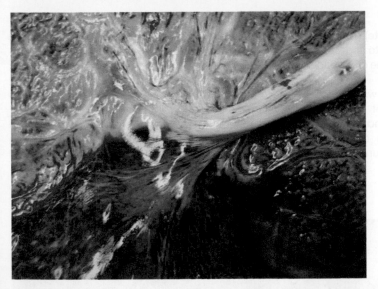

Fig. 10. The hemorrhage adjacent to the cord is located between the amnion and chorion. This is usually an artifact of placental delivery when the cord is pulled too vigorously. This cord also shows a web in which the amnionic attachment to the cord is a few centimeters above the chorionic plate. If there is rupture of velamentous vessels, the blood is also found subamniotic.

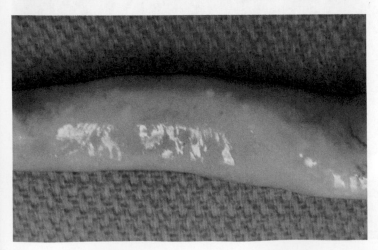

Fig. 11. Examination of the umbilical cord surface in cases of severe amniotic sac infections may reveal minute or large yellow-white foci. These are microabscesses and virtually always indicate Candida infection. A fungal stain is usually necessary to demonstrate the organisms histologically. This lesion is only seen on the cord.

Fig. 12. Note the white band from the 2-o'clock to 4-o'clock positions. This uncommon finding represents necrotic cellular debris with calcification. Such necrotizing funisitis apparently results from more chronic amniotic sac infections. The 3 vessels and the cord are of similar size and cannot be grossly identified.

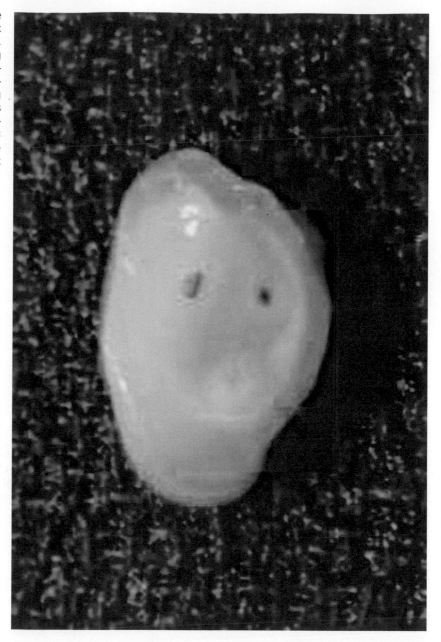

artery leads to a characteristic barber pole appearance (**Fig. 14**). The only source of nutrition to the umbilical vessels is the blood flowing within them. If a vessel is completely blocked, the muscle dies and degenerating hemoglobin leaks into Wharton jelly. This is only possible with an artery as complete occlusion of the vein is lethal.

FETAL SURFACE AND PERIPHERAL MEMBRANES

The peripheral membranes and fetal placental surface are continuous, and most processes are seen in both. The layer of membrane closest to the fetus is amnion. Peripheral, closer to the

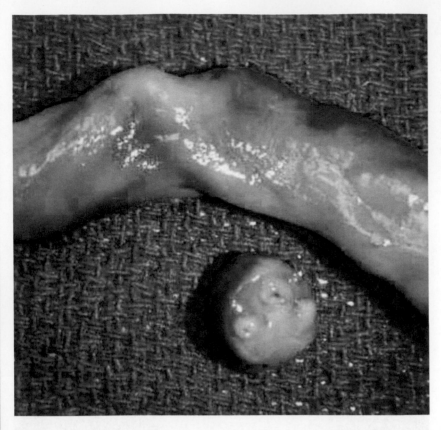

Fig. 13. With prolonged meconium exposure, the umbilical cord may become stained. The diffusion of meconium into Wharton jelly can be seen in the cross-section of cord. Necrosis of muscle cells in the vessels may occur in this setting. Note the normal 3 vessels in the cord.

uterine wall, is the chorion, which is minimal on the peripheral membranes but is continuous with all the villous tissue. The remnant of the yolk sac lies between the amnion and chorion (**Fig. 15**).

There is close proximity of the surface membranes to the maternal blood of the intervillous space, whereas the peripheral membranes abut the decidua and its blood vessels. This relationship

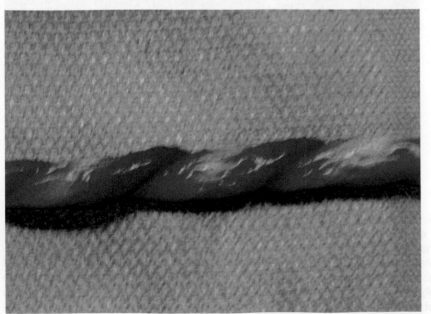

Fig. 14. The spiraling red line follows the course of one umbilical artery. There was complete thrombosis of this artery. This led to death of the muscle wall with subsequent pigment leakage.

Fig. 15. The round yellow nodule is the remnant of the yolk sac, which lies between the amnion and chorion but is not attached to either layer. They can be found in many placentas, usually near the edge of the placenta or on the membranes. Adjacent to the yolk sac is a rim of circummargination, fibrin deposition marking the edge of the vascular plate. The membranes are smooth, without a ridge. It is common to have a portion of the placental perimeter show circummargination.

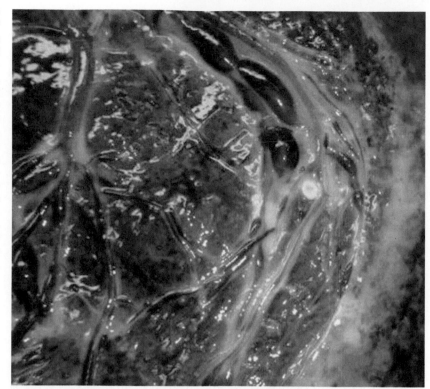

permits maternal cells access to the membranes. A variable amount of deciduas is attached to the membranes and maternal floor. This is where maternal vascular lesions are potentially found. The roll is a good place to look for these and extra sections may be rewarding in such cases.

Deposits of fibrin from the maternal circulation and thrombosis are common beneath the fetal surface. As pregnancy progresses, the amounts of these materials generally increase. Subchorionic thrombi eventually become compacted fibrin. In the presence of abundant fibrin, the trophoblastic X cells proliferate and may become cystic, either on the fetal surface or within the parenchymal septae. Although most cysts are only a few centimeters in diameter, they are occasionally much larger and may show hemorrhage. Similar lesions are seen within placental septae (**Fig. 16**). Cysts do not have any significant intrinsic pathology. Large nodular ubchorionic hematomas, sometimes called Breus moles, are seen in both liveborns and spontaneous abortions. Unusually thick layers of subchorionic hemorrhage can be associated with chronic bleeding and prematurity.

The membranes normally insert at the peripheral margin of the villous tissue, which is usually the outer limit of the vascular plate. Extrachorial

placentation exists when villous tissue extends beyond the vascular plate. This takes two forms, which often occur together. In circumvallation, there is a redundant, doubled-back membrane fold with enclosed debris and old hemorrhage at the point of membrane insertion (**Figs. 17**). In circummargination, there is a small ridge of fibrin where the membranes contact the extended placental surface (see **Fig. 14**). Circummargination is not believed to lead to clinical problems, but prematurity and chronic bleeding are associated with circumvallation. The origin of extrachorial placentation is unclear. Suggestions include abnormal implantation, secondary growth lines, marginal separation, and loss of amniotic fluid pressure.

Small nodules on the amniotic surface are either amnion nodosum or squamous metaplasia. Squamous metaplasia is considered a normal variant, whereas amnion nodosum is strongly associated with longstanding oligohydramnios, a setting in which pulmonary hypoplasia commonly develops (**Fig. 18**). Occasionally the amnion ruptures before delivery. The resulting bands of amnion can entrap and disrupt fetal tissues, leading to defects, including amputations, clefts, and constrictions. The denuded chorionic plate may be adherent to the fetus. Oligohydramnios occurs with these

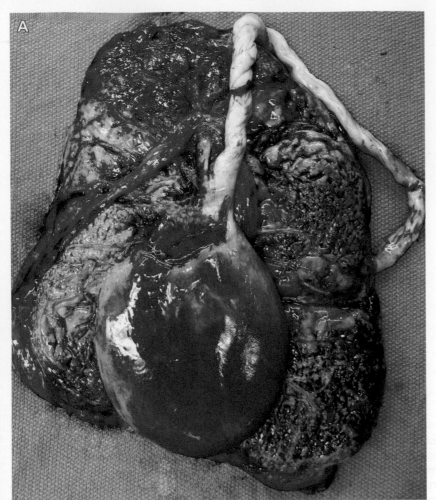

Fig. 16. (*A*) This is an unusually large subchorionic cyst. There is abundant fibrin deposition in this placenta as can be seen from the large volume of subchorionic material. The amnion has been partially peeled away showing the intrachorionic location. Hemorrhage may occur in the cysts. (*B*) Small cysts are also be seen in the chorion of the placental septae when there is abundant fibrin deposition.

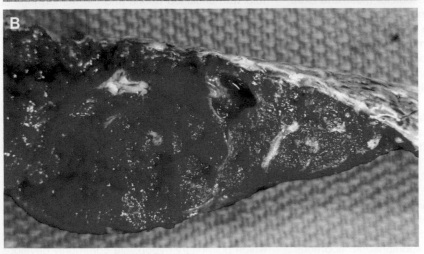

Fig. 17. (*A*) This placenta shows a wide circumvallate rim. At the edge of the vascular plate, there is a thick ridge with an overhanging lip of old hemorrhage and debris. Such placentas are generally thicker than normal. (*B*) The fetal plate is extremely small in this placenta with an unusually wide extrachorial portion. The margin is largely circummarginate.

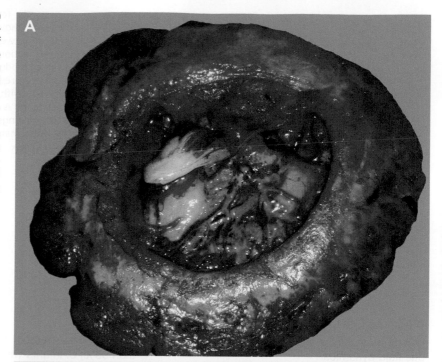

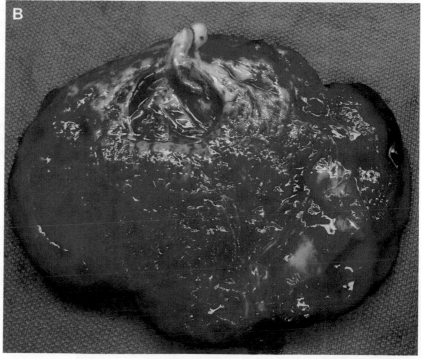

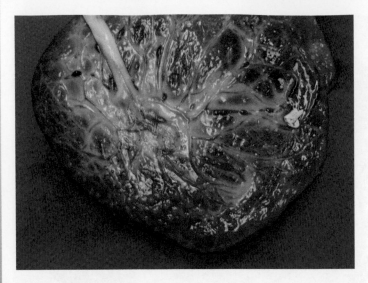

Fig. 18. The fetal surface of this preterm placenta shows tan nodules largely located between the 6-o'clock and 9-o'clock positions. This is amnion nodosum in which nodules of squames and hair, which are pressed onto the fetal surface admixed with degenerating material. This change is found only in the setting of severe, longstanding oligohydramnios. The white material at the 3-o'clock position is vernix.

lesions because the exposed chorion alters amniotic fluid dynamics.

Color and translucency of the membranes are variable, depending on pigmentation, edema, cellular content, and amount of attached decidua on the peripheral membranes (**Fig. 19**). The most frequent cause of severe surface opacity is ascending infection. The process involves maternal reaction in the surface and peripheral membranes and fetal reaction from the surface vessels and cord. Infiltrates of inflammatory cells, predominantly neutrophils, lead to the opacified appearance (**Fig. 20**). Frequently this process is clinically unsuspected. The vast majority (greater than 95%) of infants with chorioamnionitis do not become septic. There are strong indications that chorioamnionitis initiates a substantial portion of premature labor and premature rupture of the membranes.

Meconium in the amniotic fluid commonly causes green discolored membranes, particularly in late gestation. An exposed placenta can have several gross appearances (**Fig. 21**). The entire time course of histologic meconium change is not clearly established, but alterations occur within hours, not days. Many placentas in term and

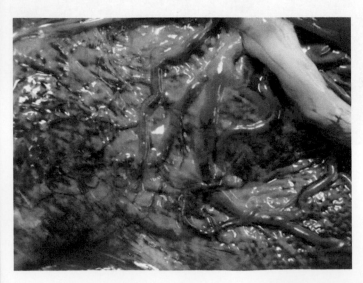

Fig. 19. There is a slight greenish opacity to the surface. It is difficult to predict the histology with this gross appearance. It is likely some meconium and/or inflammation will be found. There is abundant subchorionic fibrin and this may inhibit the maternal reaction to amniotic sac infection.

Fig. 20. The fetal surface of this severely preterm placenta is diffusely gray-green with masking of the underlying vasculature. Severe, often necrotizing chorioamnionitis have this appearance.

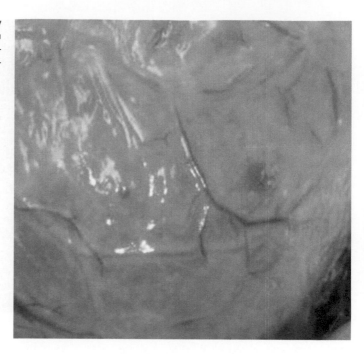

postdate pregnancies show a vaguely green color with a few pigmented macrophages in the membranes. Subsequent to affecting the membranes, meconium discolors the umbilical cord (see **Fig. 13**). All green-appearing placentas do not have meconium pigment. Extensive old hemorrhage or severe ascending infection can lead to similar coloration (**Fig. 22**) and are important

Fig. 21. The fetal surface of this placenta is bright green typical of fairly recent meconium passage. Staining rapidly moves from the amnion to sustain the chorion. This is common in terms and post-term pregnancies and is usually not associated with fetal problems.

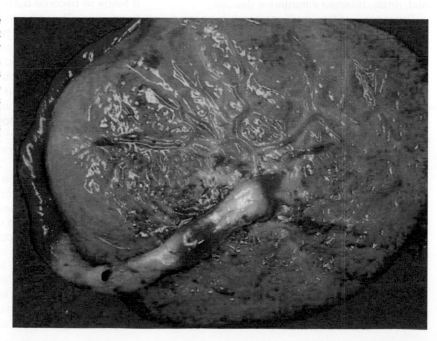

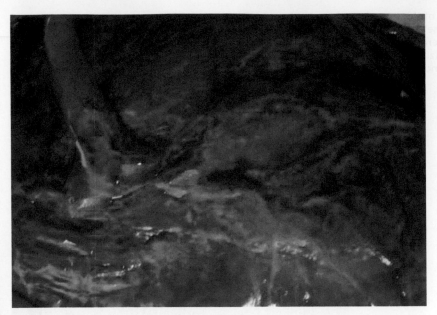

Fig. 22. A green to yellow/ brown color of the fetal surface and peripheral membranes is typical of iron pigmentation related to prolonged bleeding in or adjacent to the amniotic cavity. In severe cases, the cord also becomes stained. Chronic marginal hemorrhage and fetal disruption from amniotic bands are among the causes. Isolated yellow plaques on the membranes are usually localized areas of old retromembranous hemorrhage.

considerations in preterm pregnancies when passage of meconium is less likely. Red-brown granular thickenings and yellow areas mark old hemorrhages behind the membranes. These are common, particularly in multiple gestations, resulting from confined regions of hemorrhage in areas of decidual necrosis. Other thickenings in the membranes may represent compressed fetuses and, rarely, retained intrauterine devices.

Thrombosis of fetal surface vessels is an important observation. It occurs most commonly in fetal veins, which are always under arteries on the fetal surface (**Fig. 23**). Often thrombi are only partially occlusive of the lumen. Thrombosis is occasionally associated with inflammation or meconium but most frequently with vascular and/or cord obstruction. Calcification of vessel walls represents old thrombosis.

VILLOUS TISSUE AND MATERNAL SURFACE

The villous tissue is examined from the maternal side before and during cutting. Palpation of the placenta often reveals lesions skipped by the knife. Most villous lesions show diagnostic gross morphology. The common abnormalities are predominantly related to placental circulation, both fetal and maternal. Most disorders of significance need to be widespread in the placenta and of reasonable severity to have significant clinical consequences.

Calcification is variable but often striking feature of the maternal surface and villous tissue (**Fig. 24**). The cause is unknown and even large amounts have no recognized pathologic sequelae. Generally, calcification, like fibrin, increases with gestational age. The color of the villous tissue is largely determined by fetal hemoglobin content related both to hematocrit and total blood volume. It tends to become darker with advancing gestational age. The placentas of immature infants, who characteristically have lower hematocrits, are paler than those of term infants. Fetal vascular congestion or fetal blood loss lead to dark or light villous color. In hydrops fetalis, the placenta is large, pale, and coarse (**Fig. 25**).

True villous infarcts arise from maternal vascular problems and are common placental lesions. Most infarcts are distinctive on gross examination. These are villous regions that have lost their maternal blood supply. They are usually based on the maternal surface and have rather linear defined margins. Infarcts feel firmer than the adjacent tissue and appear granular due to the remaining collapsed villi in varying stages of degeneration. Over time, the color changes from red to white (**Fig. 26A**). Cystic change and hemorrhagic regions may be seen in infarcts. Infarction is seen most commonly at the placental margin, where there is usually less blood flow. A small (1-cm) marginal infarct in a term placenta is usually insignificant (**Fig. 27**). Central and large marginal

Fig. 23. (*A*) This placenta from a late stillbirth shows thrombosis of nearly every vein radiating out from the insertion of the cord. These are the white streaks, which pass under other vessels, and thus are veins. Chronic and acute cord compression was believed the cause of fetal demise. (*B*) This placenta is from a term liveborn infant. The cord is excessively long and shows extremely closely placed twists. There are multiple thrombi visible on the fetal surface with varying coloration, indicating they are of different ages. Fresh thrombi are red and become progressively paler over time. They are seen in both arteries and veins in this case. As in the umbilical cord, with complete obstruction, there is a stage when pigment from hemolysis spreads out from the occluded vessel.

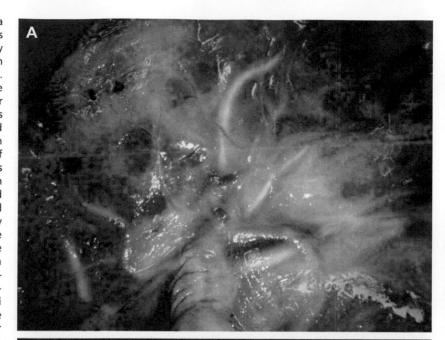

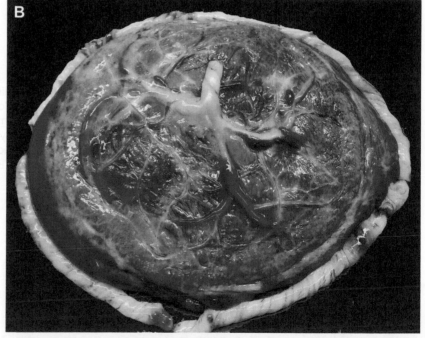

infarcts suggest, however, maternal vascular disease. Any infarction in preterm deliveries is abnormal. Examination of the entire sliced placenta is often a good means to assess the extent of villous damage (see **Fig. 26**B). Fetal problems, such as growth restriction, are often present with 15% or more infarction. Because infarcts collapse and shrink over time, they

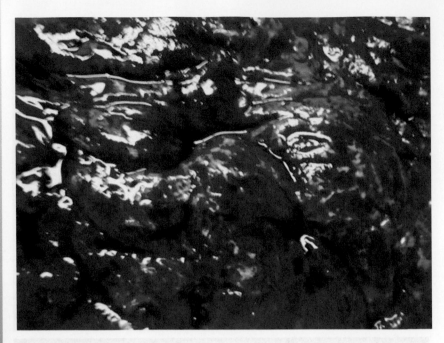

Fig. 24. The white small granular appearing areas are calcification on the maternal surface. It generally increases with gestational age. Calcification is normal and variable. It also occurs within the villous parenchyma.

represent a greater portion of villous tissue than their dimensions imply. The fetus can survive the loss of more than 50% of its placenta if the increase is gradual. Histologically, infarcts are uninteresting and should only be examined histologically as extra blocks in a heavily involved placenta. More rewarding may be sections from the maternal floor to look for decidual vascular lesions. Although common, marginal infarction is overdiagnosed by many observers. Fibrin deposition and necrotic decidua at the edge may be confusing (see **Fig. 27**B). Even occasional small

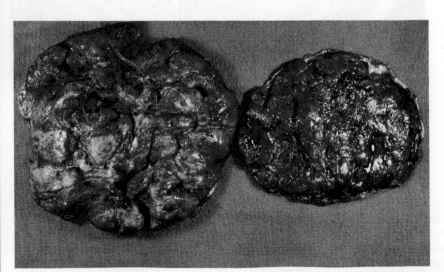

Fig. 25. A normal term placenta is present on the right with a premature hydropic placenta on the left. Note the marked increase of placental size and thickness as well as pallor in the hydropic placenta. Villous color is largely related to fetal hematocrit and amounts of blood in the placenta. With severe fetal anemia, the placenta may be almost white.

Fig. 26. (*A*) Infarcts of 2 different ages are noted in this small, totally infarcted placenta associated with a fetal demise. The paler more central infarct is older than the marginal fresh lesion. Where the maternal surface is intact, other geographic white areas of old infarct can be seen. (*B*) Cross-sections from this entire placenta are laid out to enable assessment of the percentage of the placenta involves by either infarcts or retroplacental hemorrhage.

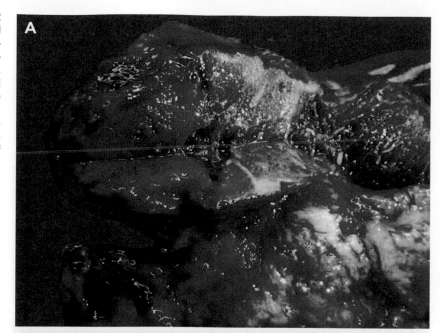

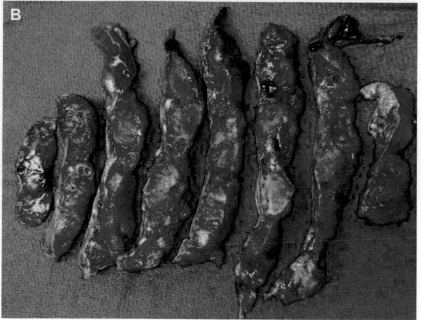

(less than 0.5 cm) central infarcts are physiologically insignificant in most cases and the extremely small ones (1–3 mm) do not warrant individual description.

Blood clots on the maternal surface of the placenta are caused by bleeding from decidual vessels in areas of premature placental separation (**Fig. 28**A). Trauma, hypertensive disorders, chorioamnionitis, smoking, and cocaine use have been associated with retroplacental hemorrhage. It is preferable to use descriptive terms for this process rather than abruptio placenta, a clinical

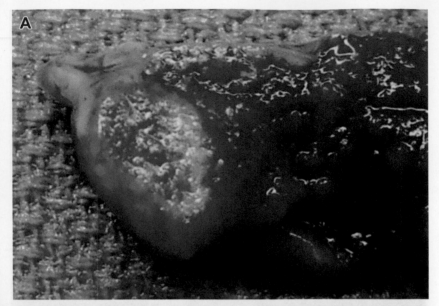

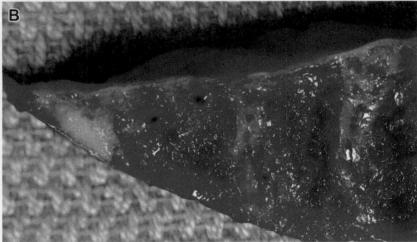

Fig. 27. (A) This true marginal infarct is clearly demarcated and has a granular appearance, as seen in this example. The white color indicates it is old. (B) The firm white shiny region at the margin of the placenta is not an infarct although it is fairly sharply defined from the adjacent villous tissue. This is likely fibrin deposition. This is often increased at the placental margin and many marginal white firm lesions are not true infarcts. Other probable fibrin deposits are in nearby villous areas.

expression implying pain and bleeding. Although some retroplacental hemorrhages correspond to clinical abruptio placenta, many grossly identified hematomas are unsuspected. It is critically important to have clinical history available at the time of examination in these situations. Recent and at times massive placental separations often show little, if any, gross or histologic change. They appear to be a normally separated placenta. Excessive blood clot received with a specimen may be the first and sometimes only clue to retroplacental hemorrhage. Most genuine fresh retroplacental hemorrhages are at least slightly adherent to the maternal surface compared with gelatinous postpartum clot. This is harder to distinguish in a fixed placenta. The gross morphology of retroplacental hemorrhage depends on the duration and degree of blood trapping. When bleeding is contained behind the placenta, the villous tissue becomes compressed by clot. If the pregnancy

Fig. 28. (*A*) The maternal surface of this placenta shows a large well-formed fresh clot, which was minimally adherent and fit within a slightly depressed area. (*B*) On cross-section, depression can better be seen. This is a fresh lesion because there is no clear infarction present. The reddened villi (*arrow*) suggest early infarction and are the oldest part of the lesion.

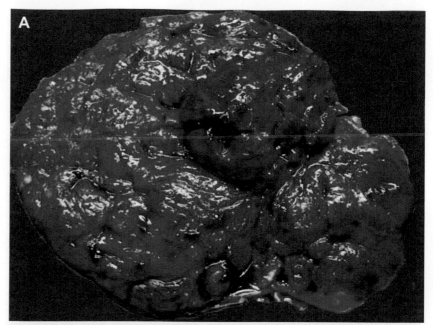

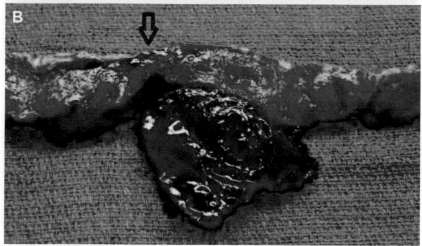

continues, the separated area infarcts because its blood supply has been lost. Lesions may be subtle on the maternal surface and better seen on cross-section. Blood and tissue degenerate and lesions become paler with time (**Fig. 29**). The exact time course for these placental changes is unknown. If the blood has a means of egress, villous tissue may not be compressed. The blood comprising the clots is largely maternal, occasionally with some fetal bleeding. Retroplacental hematomas occur both centrally and at the margin of the placenta and overlap villous tissue. If placental delivery is delayed or incomplete, fresh retroplacental hemorrhage with slightly adherent blood clot and villous collapse may be seen. This has no implications for an infant. True marginal hemorrhage also generally has no fetal effects. It is peripheral, with the aggregate of blood extending

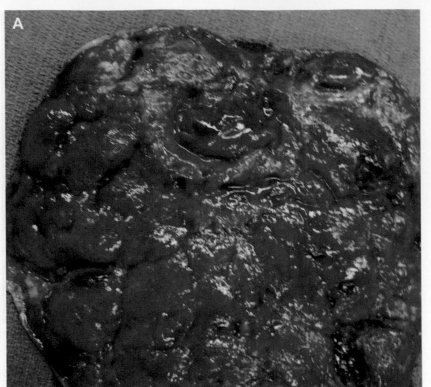

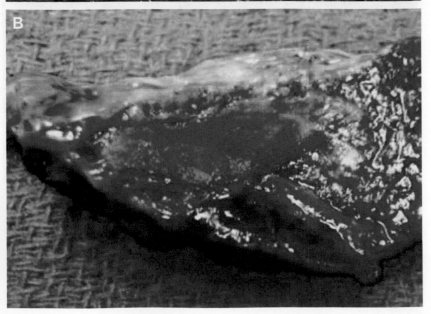

Fig. 29. (A) The brown depressed gelatinous appearing area in the upper part of the placenta is an area of old hemorrhage, a premature placental separation, which occurred some days before delivery. Old infarcts are also present away from this region at the 4 o'clock and 8 o'clock positions. (B) On cross-section of the lesion, overlying infarct can be seen. It is losing its red color as the blood is degenerating.

onto the membranes, not separating the placenta. This is a fundamentally different process, related to the marginal sinus.

Intervillous thrombi occur in the intervillous space in central areas of the placenta. The earliest thrombi are fresh red clots, which progress through laminated thrombi to old white lesions (Fig. 30). No true organization occurs. Intervillous thrombi contain both fetal and maternal red blood cells. They are seen more frequently in hydrops and other conditions with large friable placentas. The cause of these lesions is not clear but may relate to coagulation at sites of villous damage and fetal bleeding. Infarction may be present as a rim adjacent to intervillous thrombi, which apparently interfere with local villous blood supply. Such associated infarction does not imply maternal vascular disease. Intervillous thrombi may also be present at the base of the placenta, where they do not imply premature placental separation.

Localized areas of perivillous fibrin deposition are seen in virtually all mature placentas and show an irregular lacelike pattern (Fig. 31). Although the entrapped villi eventually die, small amounts of fibrin deposition are not generally thought to be related to fetal or maternal disease, apparently originating from turbulence in the maternal circulation. There are recognized disorders in which fibrin deposition is markedly increased.

Avascular villi imply interruption of the fetal blood supply. After fetal demise, the entire placenta undergoes this change if delivery does not occur. It does not infarct because maternal perfusion continues. Occlusion of only part of the fetal circulation, as with thrombosis, leads to zones of

Fig. 30. A layered lesion is present in this section of a fixed placenta. The lesion is shiny and without granularity. This is the typical location and appearance of an intervillous thrombus, generally an incidental finding. The pallor of the lesion suggests it is of some duration as much of the blood has degenerated.

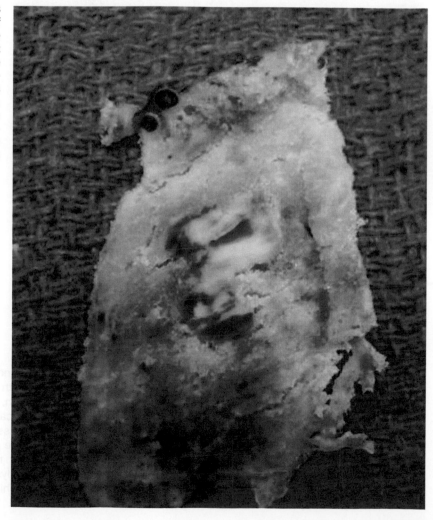

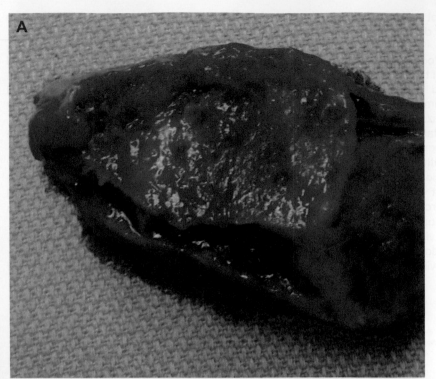

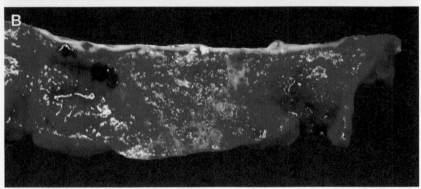

Fig. 31. (*A*) Fibrin deposition near the margin shows the typical lacy appearance with entrapped villous tissue. Fibrin is white, shiny, and nongranular. The area is clearly less deformable than the adjacent tissue. (*B*) Localized fibrin deposition may become quite dense. The slightly irregular borders, marked shine, and interior villous tissue differentiate it from an old infarct.

avascular villi, often recognizable grossly (**Fig. 32**). More localized disruptions in fetal circulation from villitis also result in avascular villous regions. This likely takes days to weeks to develop.

Other less common entities occasionally are seen. Chorangiomas are hamartomas, hemangiomas of the placenta, and occur in approximately 1% of pregnancies. These lesions commonly occur under the chorionic plate (**Fig. 33**) and have a variety of appearances, depending on vessel size, perfusion, and viability. Chorangiomas are often confused with other gross lesions. In cases of fetal infection, one may find isolated abscesses with the typical yellow necrotic appearance within the villous tissue (**Fig. 34**). Yellow, soft tissue at the base of the placenta could be infection but is more likely necrotic decidua. Large areas of mesenchymal dysplasia also are apparent on gross examination. This process is discussed in depth in another article.

Fig. 32. In this fixed piece of villous tissue, there is a pale region in the midportion of the placenta. This area has generally the same soft texture as other villous tissue. Such pale areas correspond to areas of avascular villi on histology, usually from fetal thrombotic processes.

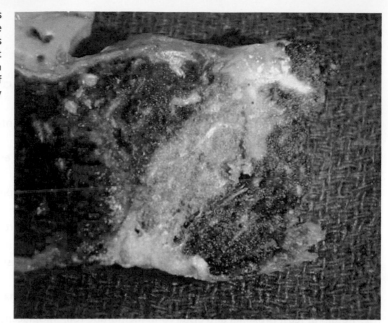

Fig. 33. The fleshy round mass under the umbilical cord is a chorangioma, a vascular hamartoma of the placenta. The appearance varies markedly depending on the viability and vascularity of the lesion. A large portion of this lesion is necrotic with focal calcifications.

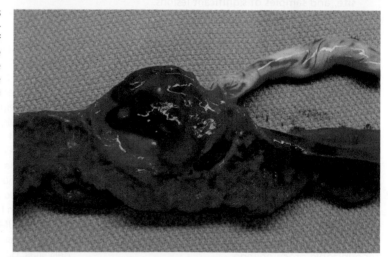

Fig. 34. Section of villous tissue shows a discrete yellow area, which appears completely necrotic. Hematogenous dissemination of fetal or maternal infection may lead to abscesses and microabscesses scattered within the villous tissue. Listeria was the cause here, but other organisms (eg, mycobacterium tuberculosis) can also cause this change.

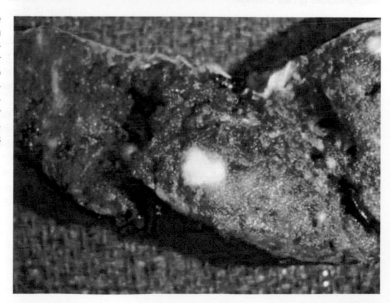

Key Points
STEPS IN THE GROSS EXAMINATION OF PLACENTAS

1. Note condition and contents of container and assess overall configuration for unusual features, which require special attention.

2. Evaluate length, twist, and insertion of umbilical cord and cut for evaluation of vessels at least 3 cm from fetal surface.

3. Evaluate fetal surface for thrombi, fibrin deposition, color, and opacity. Assess color, thickness, and completeness of peripheral membranes and note rupture site.

4. Make a jellyroll from peripheral membranes, including rupture area, and remove other membrane from the margin of placenta.

5. Palpate parenchyma and assess maternal surface for completeness, color, calcification, blood clot, and other lesions.

6. Cut the maternal surface at 2-cm intervals to evaluate parenchyma and look for additional lesions.

7. Retain at least proximal and distal cord, membrane roll, midplacental slice, including cord insertion site, and samples of significant lesions.

SUMMARY

The major gross processes commonly found in the placenta have been outlined previously. Many cord, membrane, and villous lesions are described. Experience makes most of these processes readily identifiable on inspection. Such thoughtful gross examination of a placenta before histologic sectioning optimizes the histologic interpretation through appropriate choice of areas to sample. The availability of clinical information and reason for submission is critically important to all examinations because some processes, such as premature separation, may have little recognizable gross change.

REFERENCES

1. Kaplan CG. Examination procedures. Color atlas of gross placenta pathology. 2nd edition. New York: Springer Science+Business Media; 2007. p. 1–11.
2. Yetter JF. Examination of the placenta. Am Fam Physician 1998;57(5):1045–54.
3. Dimenstein IB. A pragmatic approach to formalin safety in anatomical pathology. Lab Med 2009; 40(12):740–6.
4. Baergen RN. Macroscopic evaluation of the second and third trimester placenta. Manual of benirschke and kaufmann's pathology of the human placenta.

2nd edition. New York: Springer Science+Business Media; 2011. p. 25.
5. Molteni RA, Stys SJ, Battaglia FC. Relationship of fetal and placental weight in human beings: fetal/placental weight ratios at various gestational ages and birth weight distributions. J Reprod Med 1978; 21(5):327–34.
6. Perry IJ, Beevers DG, Whincup PH, et al. Predictors of ratio of placental weight to fetal weight in multi-ethnic community. BMJ 1995;310(6977):436–9.
7. Naeye RL. Do placental weights have clinical significance? Hum Pathol 1987;8(4):387–91.
8. Thompson JMD, Irgens LM, Skjaerven R, et al. Placenta weight percentile curves for singleton deliveries. BJOG 2007;114(6):715–20.
9. Pinar H, Sung CJ, Oyer CE, et al. Reference values for singleton and twin placental weights. Pediatr Pathol Lab Med 1996;16(6):901–7.
10. Salafia CM, Yampolsky M, Misra DP, et al. Placental surface shape, function, and effects of maternal and fetal vascular pathology. Placenta 2010;31(11): 958–62.
11. Salafia CM, Yampolsky M, Shlakhter A, et al. Variety in placental shape: when does it originate? Placenta 2012;33(3):164–70.
12. Machin GA, Ackerman J, Gilbert-Barness E. Abnormal umbilical cord coiling is associated with adverse perinatal outcomes. Pediatr Dev Pathol 2000;3(5):462–71.

Monozygotic Twinning

Kurt Benirschke, MD

KEYWORDS

- Frequency of MZ twinning • Placentation (monochorionic vs dichorionic)
- Twin-to-twin transfusion syndrome (TTTS) • Irregular splitting of embryoblasts • Acardiac twins
- Conjoined twins • Laser ablation surgery for TTTS

ABSTRACT

This article discusses pathologies found in monozygotic twinning. Detailed information is provided regarding the development during monozygotic twin formation: embryo development, twin-to-twin transfusion syndrome, acardiac twinning, vanishing twins, conjoined twins, and Beckwith-Weidmann syndrome twins. An algorithm describing the approach for identifying pathology in a placenta with multiple pregnancies is presented.

When a placenta is received of multiple pregnancies, it is best to follow the algorithm shown here:

Algorithm for

GROSS EXAMINATION IN MULTIPLE PREGNANCIES

> *Placenta of multiple pregnancy*

> *Identify number of gestations*

> *Label the umbilical cords*

> *Identify the layers that make up the "dividing membranes"*

> *Identify and describe the communicating blood vessels in the surface of the placenta*

> *This may require injection with milk or other liquid*

> *Prepare and label the sections of each placenta*

> *Determine the number of blood vessels in each umbilical cord*

OVERVIEW

Multiple gestations fall into 2 major categories:

1. Dizygotic (DZ) gestations
2. Monozygotic (MZ) pregnancies

In general, DZ gestations are either inherited (higher follicle-stimulating hormone levels, as in Nigerians, for instance), or they increase with advancing maternal age. Approximately two-thirds of multiple gestations are DZ.

MZ gestations make up approximately one-third of multiple pregnancies and their underlying cause is as yet unknown. The differences between dichorionic and monochorionic twin placentas can generally be diagnosed sonographically.

This discussion is devoted solely to MZ gestations.

DEVELOPMENT OF MONOZYGOTIC TWINNING

MZ twinning occurs spontaneously and, basically, takes place for unknown reasons. Only in the nine-banded armadillo (*Dasypus* spp) is monozygosity the rule and in these animals it results in identical quadruplets. It has also recently been reported that the frequency of MZ twinning is increased in artificial reproductive technology (ART) but the cause is not yet identified; it may relate to the prolonged culture in vitro of the blastocyst. Steinman[1] has suggested that, because the culture media contain chelating agents, "splitting" of embryoblasts occurs because cell adhesion depends on the presence of calcium ions.

In general, MZ twins can only occur during the first 2 weeks of development, before an embryonic axis has been formed. The later it occurs, the more likely conjoined twins develop and, eventually, it becomes impossible to twin. Conversely, before

Disclosure: No commercial company is discussed nor are financial interests obtained.
Department of Pathology, UCSD Medical Center, University of California San Diego, 200 West Arbor Drive, San Diego, CA 92103, USA
E-mail address: kbenirschke@ucsd.edu

Surgical Pathology 6 (2013) 27–32
http://dx.doi.org/10.1016/j.path.2012.11.006
1875-9181/13/$ – see front matter © 2013 Elsevier Inc. All rights reserved.

surgpath.theclinics.com

---

a blastocystic cavity has developed during tubal transport of the morula, MZ twins result in having a dichorionic placenta. The most problematic MZ twins from a clinical perspective are those with monochorionic placentation, and these tend to occur between days 3 and 9 after fertilization. Monoamnionic twins are likely to result and after the yolk sac forms monamnionic twins with one yolk sac develops and later, conjoined twins occur (**Fig. 1**).

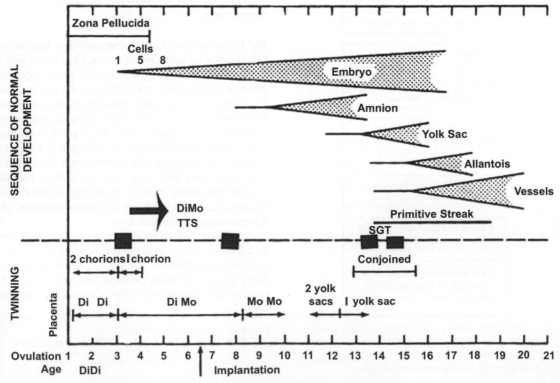

Fig. 1. Diagram displaying the first 20 days of placental and fetal development.

TWIN-TO-TWIN TRANSFUSION SYNDROME

Dichorionic MZ twins have either separate or fused placentas and are not discussed further.[2,3] Monochorionic MZ twins are the most problematic twins because they often (10%–15%) develop TTTS, and this type of placentation may also result in the formation of an acardiac twin.

Monochorionic twins are nearly always MZ with only rare exceptions recorded.[2,3] The first investigator to clearly define the vasculature of placentas and to elucidate the cause of the TTTS was Friedrich Schatz,[4] who demonstrated unequivocally the occurrence of arteriovenous connections (AVs) that allow blood to flow from the donor twin to the recipient twin through a shared cotyledon of the placenta (the so-called third circulation). In the recipient twin, cardiac hypertrophy develops as the result of plethora, and hydramnios results from this increased blood volume and excessive urination, including renal size differences. Naeye[5] defined the substantial differences of the development of many organs in these so-called identical twins. The donor twin thus becomes the stuck twin as a result of anhydramnios. Many such anastomoses may exist in a single placenta and they may even lead into different directions. Generally (but not always), a sizable artery-to-artery connection prevents the transfusion syndrome from developing.[6]

THERAPY FOR TTTS

More recently, DeLia and colleagues[7] have shown that it is feasible to occlude these AV connections by a specific laser therapy that allows thrombosis to occur in the connecting AV shunts. This therapy is now widely used and generally cures the symptomatology of the syndrome; it is summarized by Quintero.[8] Having examined many such placentas after laser ablation, I have found that the subsequent infarction of villous tissue that follows the thrombosis of surface blood vessels most often occurs only in a small, subchorionic area (Fig. 2). It is

Fig. 2. Diagram indicating why the postlaser villous infarction may be only superficial.

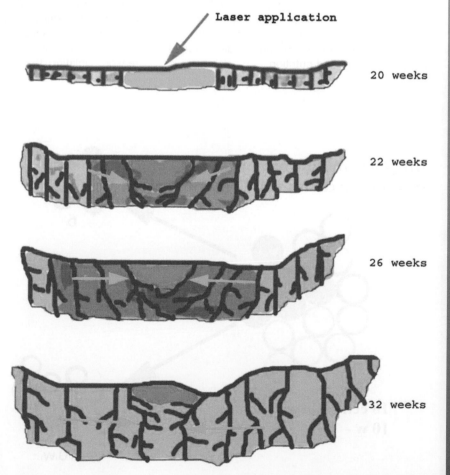

Laser application

20 weeks

22 weeks

26 weeks

32 weeks

subsequently undermined by normally perfused villous tissue. The 30-day survival of twins has been evaluated by Chmait and colleagues.[9] They found 1 twin to survive in 94% and both twins in 73%, a better survival than occurs if the twins had been let alone and not undergone laser therapy.

GROSS PATHOLOGY IN TTTS

One aspect of the TTTS is that the umbilical cords are frequently inserted abnormally; this is especially true of donor twins. Naturally, this unusual cord insertion in TTTS is also associated with a smaller placental share in the vascular distribution of the twin placenta. I have compared normal cord insertions of singletons and twins with TTTS previously and found that velamentous and marginal cord insertions are more common in donor twins.[10] The reasons for this development are not clear but it is possible that unequal splitting has a basic role in this unequal cord insertion pattern[11] (Fig. 3); alternatively, the presumably lower blood pressure of the donor fetus allows for less placental growth.

It has recently been reported that epigenetic factors (essentially methylation of specific genes) also cause discordances among MZ twins.[12,13] This is especially true for twins during their advancing age and may be due to differences in the environment and nutrition.

DEVELOPMENT OF ACARDIAC TWINS

The mechanism for the formation of acardiac twins is different from that of other MZ twins. Although acardias occur generally in monochorionic twins (in humans—it the mechanism differs in animals like cattle), it may also result from irregular splitting of the embryoblasts.[11] The acardiac fetus depends on the presence of both an artery-to-artery and a vein-to-vein anastomosis of the surface chorionic blood vessels; that arrangement of the vasculature allows for a reversal of the fetal circulation to occur between MZ twins, called TRAP by VanAllen and colleagues.[14] Most acardiac twins' umbilical cords have a single umbilical artery because of atrophy of the second artery or for other unknown reasons. Because arterial (oxygen-deprived) blood arrives in the acardiac fetus at the iliac arteries, the legs are usually better developed in acardiac twins than is the upper body. Nevertheless, many acardiac twins have been described with good upper skeletons; some acardiac twins even have a heart, and in that case, acardiac represents a misnomer. By and large, liver tissue is absent. Karyotypic analysis has commonly shown that acardiac twins are truly MZ twins and have the same karyotype as co-twins. It is possible that the presence of an acardiac twin pregnancy leads to congestive heart failure in the donor of the syndrome. For that reason, ablating the umbilical cord of acardiac

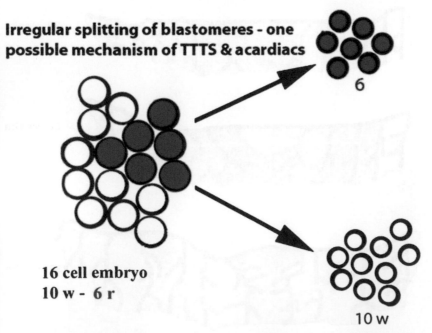

Irregular splitting of blastomeres - one possible mechanism of TTTS & acardiacs

6

16 cell embryo
10 w - 6 r

10 w

Fig. 3. Proposed irregular splitting of embryoblasts.

twins has been widely accepted, which leads to more normal development of co-twins. Ablation of the cord is accomplished by laser severance, insertion of a coil into one of the vessels, or diathermy.

DEVELOPMENT OF CONJOINED TWINS

Conjoined twins have a monoamnionic twin placenta and variable, combined or duplicated, umbilical cords. Spencer,[15] who has studied more conjoined twins than anybody, suggested that fusion of formerly split embryos was the principal mechanism to explain even the most unusual combinations of conjoined twins. Alternatively, Spemann was able to split early *Triturus* embryos partially and thus produced conjoined twins[16]; he used a hair to separate some embryoblasts in this effort (see De Robertis[16]). The placentas of conjoined twins usually have a markedly intermingled vasculature; it may be composed of a single disk when a Y-shaped umbilical cord exists.

Chimerism may be 1 of 2 kinds[17]:

1. Blood chimerism can develop from fusion of blood vessels in DZ twins.
2. Complete chimerism (so-called whole-body chimerism) may result from the fusion of 2 sets of blastomeres, either from split identical twin embryos or from DZ embryos (**Fig. 4**).

The latter type of chimerism is especially common or at least more visible in tricolored cats, and the former type occurs regularly in the usually DZ marmoset monkeys. Whole-body chimerism has been reported in several human singletons whose genitalia were ambiguous because of the fusion of male and female embryos.

DEVELOPMENT OF VANISHING TWINS

Vanishing twins occur either as a rare result of the TTTS or they may develop spontaneously in the twinning process. It is a common observation when examining placentas. A macerated, shriveled, and occasionally calcified fetus may be found. Often the membranes are severely degenerated[10] and it may be impossible to identify whether there was a dichorionic or monochorionic twin placenta. The question of whether the survivor of the twins has significant handicaps was answered in a large study by Anand and colleagues,[18] who concluded that no significant changes had been observed in survivors.

MONOZYGOTIC TWINNING AND BECKWITH-WIEDEMANN SYNDROME

The Beckwith-Wiedemann syndrome occurs considerably more frequently in female MZ twins than expected (Weksberg and colleagues[19]) and is due to a gene abnormality located at chromosome 11p15. The gene may have maternal disomy, be inverted, or have another abnormality and is methylated in unaffected twins. Whether this relates to irregular splitting of the embryoblasts (Machin[20]) or other anomalous behavior in early development has yet to be decided, but it may be increased in ART procedures (Maher and colleagues[21]).

Fig. 4. Formation of a DZ chimera by fusion of embryoblasts.

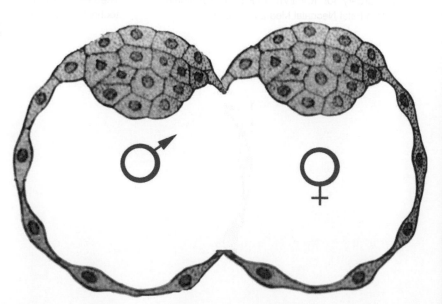

The placentas of individuals with Beckwith-Wiedemann syndrome are markedly abnormal—abnormally large and with areas of mesenchymal dysplasia.

REFERENCES

1. Steinman G. Mechanism of twinning. II. Laterality and intercellular bonding in monozygotic twinning. J Reprod Med 2001;46:473–9.
2. Quintero RA, Kontopoulos EV, Barness E, et al. Twin-twin transfusion syndrome in a dichorionic-monozygotic twin pregnancy: the end of a paradigm? Fetal Pediatr Pathol 2010;29:81–8.
3. Chmait RH, Floyd R, Benirschke K. Duplicity. Sonography suggested a twin gestation was dichorionic—and monochorionic. Am J Obstet Gynecol 2011;205: 87.e1–2.
4. Schatz F. Die Gefässverbindungen der Plazentakreisläufe eineiiger Zwillinge, ihre Entwicklung und ihre Folgen. Arch Gynakol 1884;24:337–99 and 1885;27:1–72.
5. Naeye RL. Organ abnormalities in a human parabiotic syndrome. Am J Pathol 1965;46:829–42.
6. Umur A, van Gemert MJ, Nikkels PG, et al. Monochorionic twins and twin-twin transfusion syndrome: The protective role of arterio-arterial anastomoses. Placenta 2002;23:201–9.
7. DeLia JE, Rogers JG, Dixon JA. Treatment of placental vasculature with a neodymium-yttrium-aluminum-garnet laser via fetoscopy. Am J Obstet Gynecol 1985;151:1126–7.
8. Quintero RA. Twin-twin transfusion syndrome. England: Informa UK Ltd; 2007.
9. Chmait RH, Khan A, Benirschke K, et al. Perinatal survival following preferential sequential selective laser surgery for twin-twin transfusion syndrome. J Matern Fetal Neonatal Med 2010;23:10–6.
10. Benirschke K, Kaufmann P, Baergen RN. Pathology of the human placenta. 5th edition. New York: Springer Verlag; 2006.
11. Benirschke K. The monozygotic twinning process, the twin-twin transfusion syndrome and acardiac twins. Placenta 2009;30:923–8.
12. Kato T, Iwamoto K, Kakiuchi C, et al. Genetic or epigenetic difference causing discordance between monozygotic twins as a clue to molecular basis of mental disorders. Mol Psychiatry 2005;10:622–30.
13. Tollefsbol TO. Epigenetics of aging. New York: Springer; 2009.
14. VanAllen MI, Smith DW, Shepard TH. Twin reversed arterial perfusion (TRAP) sequence: a study of 14 twin pregnancies with acardius. Semin Perinatol 1983;7:285–93.
15. Spencer R. Conjoined twins: developmental malformations and clinical implications. Baltimore: John Hopkins University Press; 2003.
16. De Robertis EM. Spemann's organizer and self-regulation in amphibian embryos. Nat Rev Mol Cell Biol 2006;7:296–302.
17. Benirschke K. Spontaneous chimerism in mammals. A critical review. Curr Top Pathol 1970;51:1–61.
18. Anand D, Platt MJ, Pharoah OD. Comparative development of surviving co-twins of vanishing twin conceptions, twins and singletons. Twin Res Hum Genet 2007;10:210–5.
19. Weksberg R, Shuma C, Caluseriu O, et al. Discordant KCNQOT1 imprinting in sets of monozygotic twins discordant for Beckwith-Wiedemann syndrome. Hum Mol Genet 2002;11:1317–25.
20. Machin GA. Some causes of genotypic and phenotypic discordance in monozygotic twin pairs. Am J Med Genet 1991;61:216–28.
21. Maher ER, Brueton LA, Bowdin SC, et al. Beckwith-Wiedemann syndrome and assisted reproductive technology. J Med Genet 2003;40:62–4.

Ascending Infection
Acute Chorioamnionitis

Füsun Gündoğan, MD[a,b], Monique E. De Paepe, MD[a,b],*

KEYWORDS

- Amniotic infection • Amniotic fluid infection syndrome • Ascending infection • Funisitis
- Chorionic vasculitis • Eosinophilic/T-cell vasculitis

ABSTRACT

Acute chorioamnionitis is a major cause of spontaneous preterm birth, accounting for more than 40% of deliveries complicated by preterm premature rupture of membranes or preterm labor. In the majority of cases, especially in preterm births, acute chorioamnionitis is caused by ascending polymicrobial infection. Recent evidence suggests that in some cases acute chorioamnionitis may have a noninfectious cause. In addition to the nonspecific patterns of conventional acute chorioamnionitis, this article describes characteristic inflammatory patterns indicative of a specific infectious cause. Several inflammatory entities of putative immunologic (noninfectious) etiology are addressed, including eosinophilic/T-cell vasculitis and chronic chorioamnionitis.

OVERVIEW

Acute chorioamnionitis is the most common pathologic condition identified after spontaneous preterm birth, especially after early preterm birth (less than 35 weeks' gestation).[1] The definition of acute chorioamnionitis varies according to key diagnostic criteria (**Box 1**). The diagnosis of clinical chorioamnionitis is based on the presence of characteristic clinical signs, including fever, uterine fundal tenderness, maternal tachycardia (greater than 100/min), fetal tachycardia (greater than 160/min), and foul amniotic fluid.[2] Histologic chorioamnionitis, the topic of this article, is defined by pathologic findings of acute inflammation on microscopic examination of the placental chorioamnion and umbilical cord.

Key Points
ACUTE CHORIOAMNIONITIS

1. Histologic chorioamnionitis is characterized by the presence of neutrophils in well-defined chorioamnionic compartments of the placenta and/or in the umbilical cord.

2. In the majority of cases, especially in preterm births, acute chorioamnionitis is linked to ascending polymicrobial infection.

3. The infectious organisms (or noninfectious factors eliciting inflammation) induce a stereotypical sequence of maternal and fetal inflammatory reaction patterns.

4. The clinical significance of acute chorioamnionitis correlates with the magnitude and progression of these maternal and fetal inflammatory responses, which can be estimated from the extent and anatomic location of the respective acute inflammatory reaction patterns.

5. A clinically relevant diagnostic report is expected to include a description of the specific fetal and maternal inflammatory responses involving both chorionic plate and extraplacental membranes.

6. Actual staging and grading of acute chorioamnionitis is optional.

The reported frequency of chorioamnionitis varies greatly according to diagnostic criteria (eg, clinical vs histologic chorioamnionitis), specific risk group, and gestational age.[2–4] Overall, 1% to

---

[a] Department of Pathology, Women and Infants Hospital, 101 Dudley Street, Providence, RI 02905, USA;
[b] Department of Pathology and Laboratory Medicine, Alpert Medical School of Brown University, 222 Richmond Street, Providence, RI 02905, USA
* Corresponding author. Department of Pathology, Women and Infants Hospital, 101 Dudley Street, Providence, RI 02905.
E-mail address: mdepaepe@wihri.org

Surgical Pathology 6 (2013) 33–60
http://dx.doi.org/10.1016/j.path.2012.11.002
1875-9181/13/$ – see front matter © 2013 Elsevier Inc. All rights reserved.

Box 1
Key diagnostic criteria: acute chorioamnionitis—classifications

Histologic chorioamnionitis	Microscopic evidence of acute inflammation • Chorioamnion of extraplacental membranes and/or chorionic plate • Umbilical cord
Clinical chorioamnionitis	Clinical manifestations of local and systemic inflammation • Fever (>37.5°C) • Uterine tenderness • Abdominal pain • Foul smelling vaginal discharge • Maternal and fetal tachycardia • Elevated white blood cell count
Clinical chorioamnionitis—supported by microbiology results	Positive microbial cultures from appropriately collected amniotic fluid, chorioamnion, or fetus/neonate
Clinical chorioamnionitis—supported by inflammatory biomarker profiles	Elevated levels of proinflammatory cytokines in cord blood and/or amnion • Interleukin (IL)-6, IL-8, matrix metalloproteinase (MMP), chemokine (C-X-C motif) ligand 6 (CXCL6), and others

4% of all births in the United States are complicated by chorioamnionitis.[5] Among preterm births, as many as 40% to 70% of deliveries associated with premature rupture of membranes or spontaneous labor are complicated by chorioamnionitis (clinical and histologic combined)[6] compared with 1% to 13% of term births.[3,7–9]

Risk factors for chorioamnionitis include prolonged membrane rupture, prolonged labor, multiple digital examinations with membrane rupture, group B streptococcus colonization, bacterial vaginosis, alcohol and tobacco use, meconium-stained amniotic fluid, and epidural anesthesia (reviewed by Tita and Andrews[3]). Although preterm premature (prelabor) rupture of membranes (PPROM) is a major risk factor for chorioamnionitis, PPROM and preterm labor frequently are consequences, rather than causes, of subclinical chorioamnionitis.[10] Furthermore, acute chorioamnionitis is seen both in cases of PPROM and in cases of preterm labor with intact membranes.

The pathogenesis of chorioamnionitis is multifactorial and, to some extent, gestational age dependent. In preterm infants, chorioamnionitis is most commonly caused by ascending polymicrobial bacterial infection from the lower genital tract (cervix and vagina).[5,11] The most frequent microbes associated with chorioamnionitis are the genital mycoplasmas, *Ureaplasma urealyticum* and *Mycoplasma hominis*, detected in up to 47% and 30%,

respectively, of culture-confirmed cases of chorioamnionitis.[11,12] Other common isolates in pregnancies complicated by chorioamnionitis include anaerobes, such as *Gardnerella vaginalis* and bacteroides, and aerobes, including group B streptococcus and gram-negative rods, such as *Escherichia coli*.[11]

Less common routes of infection are hematogenous or transplacental passage, iatrogenic infection associated with amniocentesis or chorionic villus sampling, and spread of infectious agents from the peritoneum via the fallopian tubes.[3] Fetoplacental infection with *Listeria monocytogenes* is generally believed due to hematogenous rather than ascending infection.[13] Although in preterm infants chorioamnionitis is typically linked to an infectious cause, several lines of evidence suggest that chorioamnionitis in low-risk term gestations and in a subset of preterm gestations may have a noninfectious, possibly immune-mediated etiology.[14] Additional proposed noninfectious causes of histologic chorioamnionitis include fetal hypoxia, amniotic fluid pH changes, meconium exposure, and other nonspecific responses.[15]

The inflammatory response associated with acute chorioamnionitis is accompanied by the release of proinflammatory cytokines and chemokines in the respective fetal and maternal compartments. The severity of placental inflammation has been shown to correlate with the concentrations of fetal/neonatal inflammatory mediators, such as IL-6, IL-8, matrix metalloproteinase-8, and CXCL6 in amniotic fluid and/or cord blood.[16–23] The potential clinical utility of amniotic fluid and other inflammatory biomarkers as proxy of the fetal inflammatory response has sparked interest in proteomic profiling of the amniotic fluid for detection or prediction of inflammation, infection, and neonatal sepsis.[24]

Acute chorioamnionitis is a major risk factor for spontaneous preterm birth. Additional consequences of acute chorioamnionitis and associated fetal inflammatory response include an increased risk for cystic periventricular leukomalacia, intraventricular hemorrhage, and cerebral palsy in preterm infants.[3,25–27] Histologic chorioamnionitis has protective effects for respiratory distress syndrome in preterm infants; however, this short-term beneficial effect is followed by increased susceptibility of the lung to subsequent postnatal injury and a predisposition for bronchopulmonary dysplasia (chronic lung disease) (reviewed by Thomas and Speer[28]). Prenatal inflammation/infection is a risk factor for early-onset neonatal sepsis, although the risk of late-onset sepsis in preterm infants may be reduced in association with histologic chorioamnionitis.[29] Several of these associations remain controversial, because the gestational age-independent effects of chorioamnionitis on neonatal outcome have become less evident with advances in neonatal care.[28]

Acute chorioamnionitis is characterized by infiltration of maternal and/or fetal neutrophils in the chorioamniotic membranes and the umbilical cord (which are usually devoid of neutrophils). Certain maternal and fetal histologic inflammatory reaction patterns have been shown to correlate with pregnancy outcome.[30–32] For instance, the presence of umbilical panvasculitis and subchorionic microabscesses may indicate an increased risk for early-onset neonatal sepsis. Other placental characteristics, such as funisitis and intense chorionic vasculitis with intravascular thrombi, may connote an increased risk for long-term neurologic impairment.[31,32] Necrotizing chorioamnionitis and/or funisitis may be indicative of long-standing infection,[32] and the presence of histologic acute chorioamnionitis, in general, may confirm the clinical suspicion of amniotic fluid infection.

Based on the reported clinicopathologic correlations between patterns of histologic chorioamnionitis and pregnancy outcome, contemporary pathology reporting of acute chorioamnionitis is expected to include a description of the types and severity of fetal and maternal histologic inflammatory responses involving both chorionic plate and extraplacental membranes. Grading and staging systems to score the severity and progression of acute chorioamnionitis have been described[33,34] but have not found universal acceptance for routine diagnostic purposes.

Finally, the absence of histologic acute chorioamnionitis does not exclude potentially serious fetal or neonatal infection. For group B streptococcus infection, a leading cause of invasive bacterial disease in the neonatal period, histologic fetoplacental inflammation is a notoriously poor indicator of perinatal infection, especially in preterm fetuses/newborns.[35]

ACUTE CHORIOAMNIONITIS: GROSS FEATURES

When sufficiently abundant, the acute inflammatory exudate collecting as component of the maternal inflammatory response may impart a dull and opaque-yellow appearance to the extraplacental membranes and the membranes covering the chorionic plate (**Fig. 1**). The chorionic vasculature may be obscured by opacification of the overlying chorionic membranes. Marked neutrophilic exudation can result in green-yellow discoloration of the membranes, similar to the staining observed after exposure of the membranes to meconium or biliverdin (as seen in association with chronic abruption). The fetal inflammatory response may be associated with induration of the chorionic plate vessels. Umbilical vasculitis and perivasculitis may result in concentric yellow-white, sometimes chalky arcs around the umbilical vessels (**Fig. 2**).

ACUTE CHORIOAMNIONITIS: MICROSCOPIC FEATURES

The neutrophil infiltration in acute chorioamnionitis progresses according to a stereotypical sequence of maternal and fetal histopathologic acute inflammatory responses. The maternal inflammatory response is characterized by infiltration of chorionic plate and membranous chorioamnion by maternal neutrophils originating from the intervillous space and vessels of the decidua capsularis, respectively. The fetal inflammatory response consists of transmigration of neutrophils (and occasionally eosinophils) from the fetal circulation through the wall of large-sized fetal vessels into chorionic plate and umbilical cord.

Current standard practice involves detailed description of placental findings using standardized diagnostic terminology and based on specific diagnostic criteria.[34] Actual staging and grading of the respective inflammatory responses is optional in daily practice but may be useful for research or other academic purposes. A proposed template for reporting of acute chorioamnionitis is shown in the **Box 2**. It is most accurate to use the term, *acute chorioamnionitis*, rather than the often-used

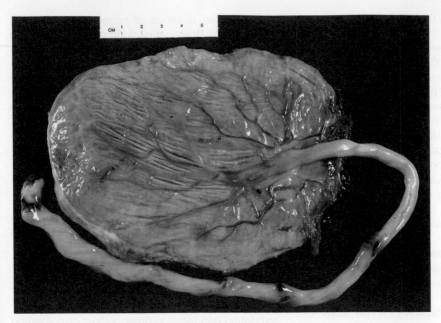

Fig. 1. Acute chorioam-nionitis. Dull and opa-que-yellow appearance of fetal surface of the placenta.

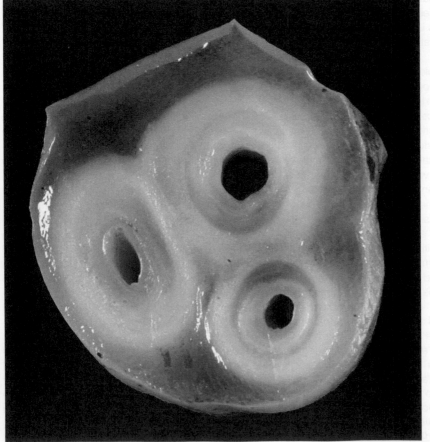

Fig. 2. Necrotizing funisi-tis. Cross-section of a cord with concentric yellow-white arcs around the vessels, composed of aggregates of necrotic inflammatory cells.

> **Box 2**
> **Acute chorioamnionitis: key points to be included in the pathology report**
>
> - Maternal inflammatory response
>   - Chorionic plate
>   - Acute subchorionitis
>   - Acute chorioamnionitis
>   - Necrotizing chorioamnionitis
>   - Extraplacental membranes
>   - Acute chorionitis
>   - Acute chorioamnionitis
>   - Necrotizing chorioamnionitis
>   - Modifiers
>   - Presence of subchorionic microabscesses
>   - Evidence of subacute (prolonged) chorioamnionitis
>   - Presence of specific microorganisms (eg, *Fusobacterium*)
> - Fetal inflammatory response
>   - Chorionic plate
>   - Chorionic vasculitis
>   - Umbilical cord
>   - Umbilical phlebitis
>   - Umbilical vasculitis with arterial involvement
>   - Umbilical panvasculitis with extension to Wharton substance (funisitis)
>   - Umbilical panvasculitis with necrotizing funisitis
>   - Modifiers
>   - Presence of peripheral funisitis with *Candida* sp
>   - Presence of occlusive/nonocclusive chorionic/umbilical thrombi

terms, *evidence of intrauterine infection* and *amniotic fluid infection syndrome*.

MATERNAL INFLAMMATORY RESPONSE

The maternal inflammatory response is assessed by evaluating the anatomic progression of (maternally derived) acute inflammatory infiltrates in the chorioamnion of extraplacental membranes and chorionic disc. In the early stage, acute subchorionitis and/or acute chorionitis, maternal neutrophils, derived from the intervillous space, accumulate in the subchorionic plate fibrin (acute subchorionitis) (Fig. 3A) and/or membranous chorionic trophoblast layer (acute chorionitis) (see Fig. 3B). A few scattered neutrophils infiltrating the lower portions of the chorionic plate and/or membranous chorionic connective tissue are allowed.

In acute chorioamnionitis, more than a few scattered maternal neutrophils are present in the connective tissues of the chorionic plate and membranous chorioamnion (Fig. 4A). In necrotizing chorioamnionitis, the amnion basement membrane is hypereosinophilic, associated with massive karyorrhexis of degenerating neutrophils and at least focal necrosis and detachment of amnionic epithelial cells (see Fig. 4B). When describing necrotizing chorioamnionitis, a distinction needs to be made between involvement of chorionic plate and extraplacental membranes only.

The severity of the maternal inflammatory response can further be described as mild to moderate (individual or small clusters of maternal neutrophils diffusely infiltrating amnion, chorionic plate, chorion laeve, and/or subchorionic fibrin [Fig. 5A, B]) or severe (presence of a continuous band of confluent chorionic neutrophils [see Fig. 5C] or the presence of microabscesses between chorion and decidua in the membranes and/or under the subchorionic plate [see Fig. 5D]).

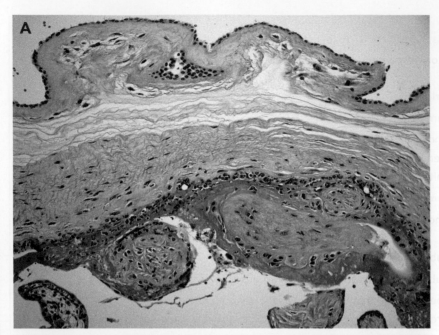

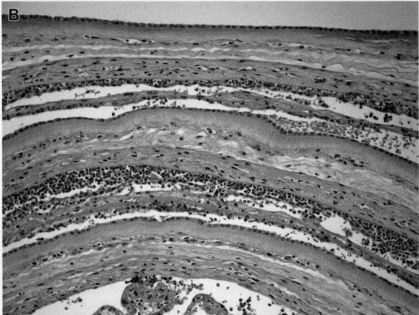

Fig. 3. Early maternal inflammatory response. The initial phase of the maternal inflammatory response is characterized by the presence of neutrophils in the subchorionic fibrin (acute subchorionitis) (*A*) and/or membranous chorionic trophoblast layer (acute chorionitis) (*B*).

FETAL INFLAMMATORY RESPONSE

The fetal inflammatory response is characterized by transmigration of fetal neutrophils from the fetal chorionic and umbilical circulation into the muscular walls of veins and arteries in the chorionic plate (chorionic vasculitis) and/or umbilical cord (umbilical vasculitis, sometimes referred to as funisitis). Fetal inflammatory response restricted to the chorionic plate vessels tends to be more common in preterm placentas, whereas involvement of umbilical vessels alone, in particular the vein, is more common at term.[36] Similar to the maternal response, the fetal inflammatory response has been shown to progress according to a specific sequence: involvement of the umbilical vein and chorionic plate vessels usually precedes that of the arteries.[33,37]

Fig. 4. Acute chorioamnionitis. After the initial phase, polymorphonuclear leukocytes continue to migrate toward the amniotic cavity. Extension of neutrophils to chorionic and amniotic stroma constitutes acute chorioamnionitis (*A*). Necrotizing chorioamnionitis is characterized by severe acute inflammation with karyorrhexis, hypereosinophilic amniotic basement membrane and at least focal necrosis of the amniotic epithelium (*B*).

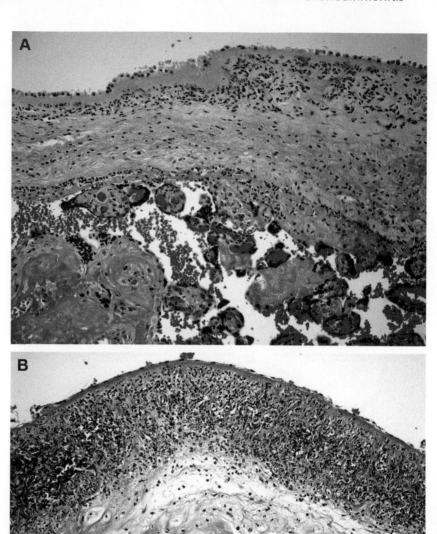

Inflammation of one or both umbilical arteries is associated with higher fetal cytokine levels and higher neonatal morbidity than inflammation of the vein only.[16,38] Furthermore, umbilical panvasculitis (vein plus arteries) is an independent risk factor for neonatal sepsis.[30] These data stress the importance of differentiating between involvement of the umbilical vein alone (phlebitis) and umbilical vasculitis with arterial involvement.[34] The term, *funisitis*, is variably used in the literature to describe inflammation of the umbilical vessels (umbilical vasculitis, vessel type unspecified) or inflammation of Wharton substance (umbilical perivasculitis). The use of this nonspecific generic term to describe the umbilical vascular inflammatory response is discouraged when used alone unless more specific descriptors are included.

In the early stages, chorionic vasculitis and/or umbilical phlebitis, fetal neutrophils are localized to the wall of chorionic plate vessels (**Fig. 6**A) or

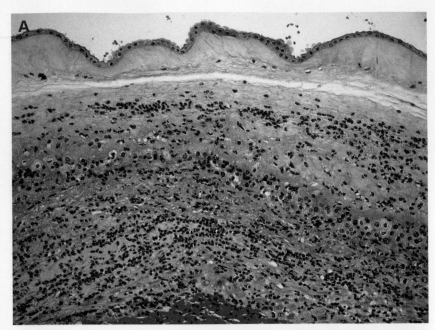

Fig. 5. Grading of maternal inflammatory response. In mild moderate chorioamnionitis, maternal neutrophils diffusely infiltrate amnion and chorion laeve (*A*) and/or chorionic plate (*B*), either individually or in small clusters.

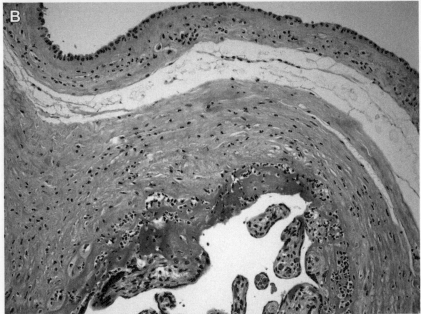

the umbilical vein (see **Fig. 6**B). In more advanced stages of fetal inflammatory response, defined by the presence of umbilical arteritis, fetal neutrophils infiltrate the wall of one or both umbilical arteries (see **Fig. 6**C), with or without involvement of the umbilical vein. A few neutrophils may be present in Wharton substance at these stages, as long as they are not aggregated in a concentric band, ring, or halo around the umbilical vessels. In umbilical panvasculitis, all 3 umbilical vessels are involved by neutrophils and infiltrates extend into Wharton substance without concentric necrosis (**Fig. 7**A). In necrotizing funisitis or concentric umbilical perivasculitis, wide layers of degenerating neutrophils and cellular debris are arranged in concentric arcs around one or more umbilical vessels (see **Fig. 7**B). This lesion, associated with longstanding infection, may undergo band-like

Fig. 5. continued, Grading of maternal inflammatory response. Presence of a continuous band of confluent chorionic neutrophils (*C*) and microabscesses in subchorionic space of the chorionic plate (*D*) are features of severe inflammation.

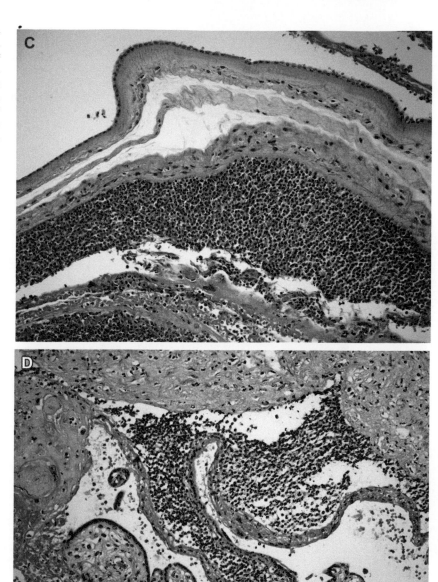

calcification resulting in chalky white arcs encircling the umbilical vessels on gross examination (barber pole lesion) (see **Fig. 2**).

In mild moderate fetal inflammatory response, scattered neutrophils infiltrate the subendothelial or intramural portions of any chorionic (or umbilical) vessel (**Fig. 8**A). In severe inflammation, there is near confluent accumulation of neutrophils in chorionic plate (or umbilical) vessels with attenuation and/or degeneration of vascular smooth muscle cells on the side facing the amniotic cavity (see **Fig. 8**B). Endothelial injury and activation may promote the formation of occlusive or nonocclusive chorionic vessel thrombi, which may occasionally embolize to the fetus. Chorionic thrombi are characterized by glassy red-blue staining,

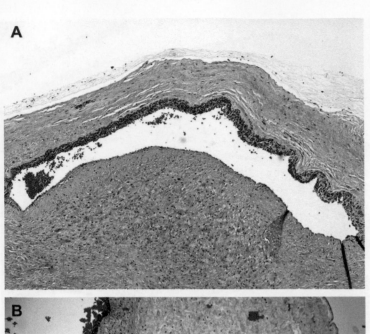

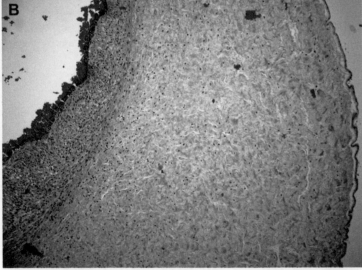

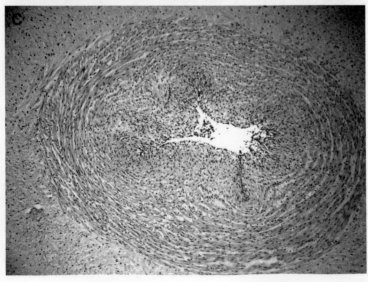

Fig. 6. Early fetal inflammatory response. Fetal neutrophils marginate and then infiltrate the chorionic vessels (*A*), umbilical vein (*B*), and later one or both umbilical arteries (*C*) in the direction of the amniotic cavity.

Fig. 7. Funisitis. In severe fetal inflammatory response, fetal neutrophils infiltrate the umbilical vasculature and expand into Wharton substance (funisitis) without forming necrotic bands (*A*). At later stages, necrotizing funisitis is defined by the presence of concentric bands around the vessels formed by degenerating neutrophils and cellular karyorrhexis (*B*).

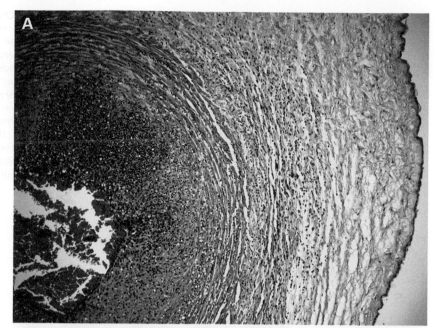

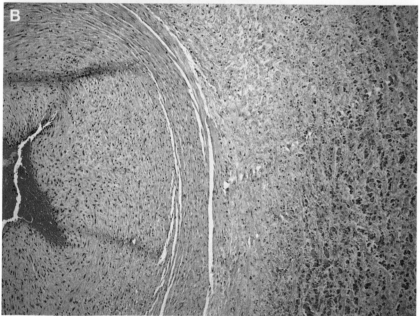

lamination, and adhesion to the vessel wall (see Fig. 8C).

IDENTIFICATION OF INFECTIOUS ORGANISMS

Placental cultures and special stains are not routinely performed in cases of acute chorioamnionitis. Acute chorioamnionitis is usually caused by a polymicrobial infection and often involves mycoplasma and anaerobic bacteria that are notoriously difficult to stain or culture. Furthermore, these ancillary studies are unlikely to influence clinical management and may be misleading if not performed correctly.[39] In selected clinical settings, such as a compromised newborn with suspected sepsis whose mother was treated with antibiotics before delivery, special stains or placental cultures may be helpful. In these cases, silver impregnation stains (Steiner, Dieterle, and Warthin-Starry) have the highest

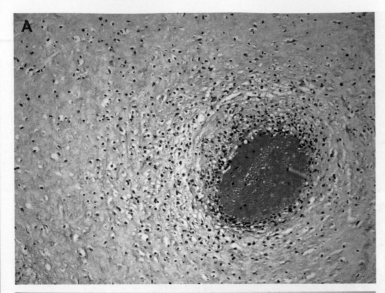

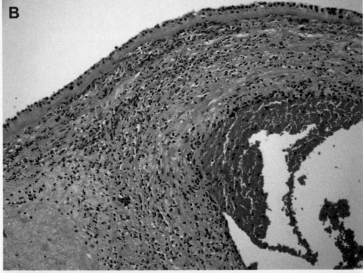

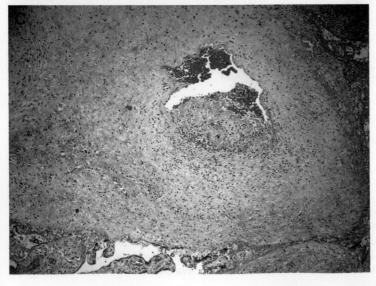

Fig. 8. Chorionic vasculitis. Transmigration of fetal neutrophils into chorionic plate vessels individually or in small clusters is defined as mild-moderate fetal inflammatory response (*A*). As in the umbilical cord, severe inflammatory response results in concentric accumulation of neutrophils and cellular debris around the chorionic vessels (*B*). Associated endothelial damage may initiate a cascade of events that results in thrombus formation (*C*).

sensitivity for demonstrating bacteria in placental tissue sections.[39] Parenthetically, the presence of bacteria within the fetal vessels of umbilical cord, chorionic plate, and/or stem villi may provide indirect evidence of fetal bacteremia, even in the absence of positive culture results.[40]

Most often, bacterial stains performed in the context of acute chorioamnionitis demonstrate a mixture of nondistinctive cocciform and bacilliform organisms. One exception is the typical histopathologic pattern seen in chorioamnionitis caused by *Fusobacterium* sp, gram-negative anaerobic bacilli associated with periodontal disease. In these cases, a characteristic meshwork of long, slender filamentous bacteria is noted along the denuded amnion (**Fig. 9**).[41,42]

ACUTE CHORIOAMNIONITIS: MATERNAL INFLAMMATORY RESPONSE-DIFFERENTIAL DIAGNOSIS

CHRONIC CHORIOAMNIONITIS

Chronic chorioamnionitis is defined by infiltration of lymphocytes in the chorioamniotic membranes (**Fig. 10A**).[43–45] Especially in poorly preserved specimens, the mononuclear cell infiltrates of chronic chorioamnionitis may resemble the neutrophil infiltrates of acute chorioamnionitis. The cause of chronic chorioamnionitis is unknown. Although subclinical amniotic fluid infection (eg, viral) remains a possibility, the frequent association of chronic

chorioamnionitis with villitis of unknown etiology and the altered chemokine profile in the amniotic fluid suggest an immunologic cause, consistent with maternal antifetal cellular rejection.[46,47] Chronic chorioamnionitis has been associated with spontaneous preterm birth, previous spontaneous abortion, and intrauterine growth restriction.

Microscopically, chronic chorioamnionitis is characterized by focal infiltration of maternally derived CD3-positive T lymphocytes in the chorioamniotic membranes and, to a lesser extent, the chorionic plate (see **Fig. 10A**). Other pathologic findings associated with this pattern of chronic chorioamnionitis include chronic villitis of unknown etiology and chronic deciduitis with plasma cells (see **Fig. 10B**).[46] In a second pattern, chronic chorioamnionitis may be accompanied by acute chorioamnionitis in the same placenta, producing an acute-on-chronic chorioamnionitis pattern.[43,46]

LAMINAR NECROSIS

Laminar necrosis of the placental membranes is a recently described histologic lesion characterized by a band of coagulative necrosis with neutrophil infiltrates at the choriodecidual interphase.[48] Laminar necrosis has been reported in placentas from pregnancies complicated by preeclampsia, PPROM, and preterm abruption. Although laminar necrosis has been speculated as linked to placental hypoxia, the exact pathogenesis and clinical significance of this somewhat controversial lesion remain undetermined.

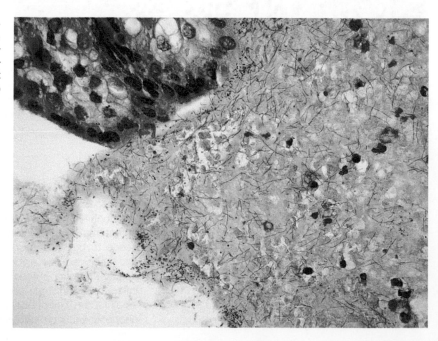

Fig. 9. Fusobacterium. Blood clot with long, slender, filamentous bacteria, which are gram-negative and consistent with *Fusobacterium* sp (Gram stain).

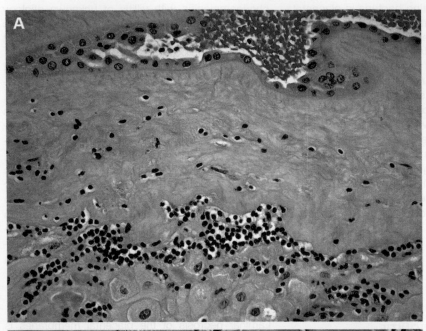

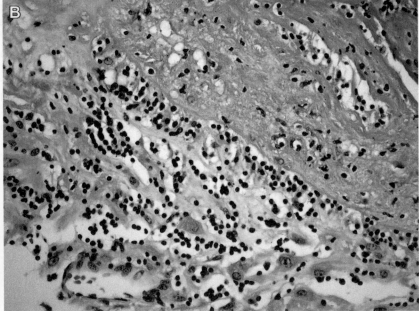

Fig. 10. Chronic chorioamnionitis. Infiltration of chorioamniotic membranes by lymphocytes (*A*) (chronic chorioamnionitis) is usually accompanied by infiltration of the decidua by lymphocytes and plasma cells (*B*) (chronic deciduitis).

ACUTE CHORIOAMNIONITIS: FETAL INFLAMMATORY RESPONSE-DIFFERENTIAL DIAGNOSIS

EOSINOPHILIC/T-CELL CHORIONIC VASCULITIS

Eosinophils can be a significant component of the fetal inflammatory response to intrauterine infection.[32,49] Presumably fetally derived eosinophils have been described in the wall of chorionic or umbilical vessels in approximately 20% of preterm births.[49] Eosinophil-rich fetal inflammatory response as a feature of conventional acute chorioamnionitis needs to be distinguished from eosinophilic/T-cell chorionic vasculitis, a poorly understood and recently described entity characterized by a fetally derived inflammatory infiltrate composed of eosinophils and small CD3+ T lymphocytes localized to the wall of chorionic and stem villous vessels.[50]

ΔΔ

Differential Diagnosis
ACUTE CHORIOAMNIONITIS

Maternal inflammatory response	
Chronic chorioamnionitis	• Lymphocytes in membranes (and chorionic plate)
	• Associated villitis of unknown cause
	• Noninfectious, likely immune mediated
Laminar necrosis	• Band of coagulative necrosis with neutrophils in membranes
	• Possibly related to placental hypoxia
Fetal inflammatory response	
Eosinophilic/T-cell chorionic vasculitis	• Eosinophils and T lymphocytes
	• Focal involvement of single chorionic vessel
	• Associated villitis of unknown etiology
	• Noninfectious, likely immune mediated
Meconium-associated vascular necrosis	• Eosinophilic cytoplasmic degeneration and rounding of vascular smooth muscle cells
	• Nuclear pyknosis
	• Occasionally associated neutrophils
	• Evidence of meconium exposure
Villitis of unknown cause with vascular involvement	• Mixed lymphocyte/macrophage infiltrate
	• May involve chorionic and stem villus vessels
	• Noninfectious, likely immune mediated
	• Associated with poor pregnancy outcome and recurrent pregnancy loss

The frequency of eosinophilic/T-cell chorionic vasculitis is reported as less than 0.1% to 0.6% of placentas examined.[50,51] Eosinophilic/T-cell chorionic vasculitis has no recognized clinical associations thus far.[51] The vasculitis seems absent before 34 weeks' gestation, similar to villitis of unknown etiology. Although the exact etiology of eosinophilic T-cell chorionic vasculitis remains unclear, a noninfectious, immunologic origin is likely.[32,51]

Microscopically, a mixed lymphoid/eosinophil infiltrate is present in the muscular wall of chorionic plate vessels (**Fig. 11**). Eosinophilic/T-cell chorionic vasculitis typically only focally involves a single chorionic artery or vein, occasionally extending into stem villous vasculature.[50] According to the original description based on a relatively small series, the inflammation characteristically radiates toward the intervillous space (in contrast to the radiation toward amniotic fluid seen in the fetal choriovascular

response to chorioamnionitis).[50] In a subsequent larger series of eosinophilic/T-cell chorionic vasculitis cases, inflammation had no predominant direction in approximately two-thirds of cases and was as likely to face the intervillous space as the amniotic cavity in the remainder.[51] Narrowing of the vascular lumen, vascular thrombosis, and vascular or villous changes of fetal vascular thrombo-occlusive disease may be present.[50,51]

Villitis of unknown etiology is seen in more than 40% of placentas with eosinophilic/T-cell chorionic vasculitis.[51] The frequency of acute inflammatory lesions (maternal or fetal inflammatory response) is not increased in placentas with eosinophilic/T-cell chorionic vasculitis.[51]

In contrast to eosinophilic/T-cell chorionic vasculitis, the eosinophil-rich vasculitis that occurs in the setting of conventional acute chorioamnionitis is usually accompanied by other histologic

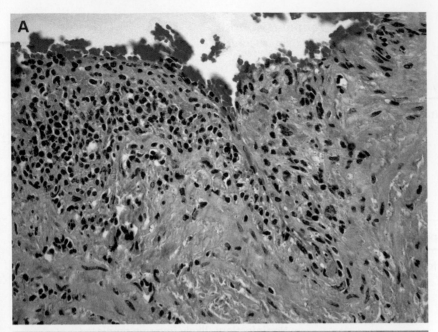

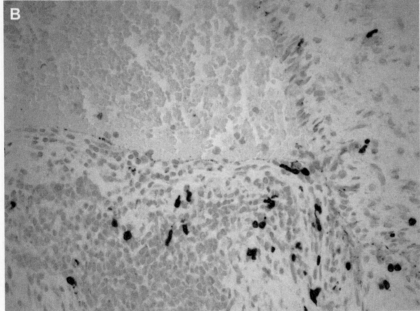

Fig. 11. Eosinophilic/T-cell chorionic vasculitis. The chorionic plate vessel is densely infiltrated by eosinophils and lymphocytes radiating toward the intervillous space (*A*). Immunohistochemical staining highlights the presence of CD3+ T lymphocytes in the inflammatory infiltrate (B: anti-CD3 immunohistochemistry with hematoxylin counterstain).

indicators of acute chorioamnionitis.[49] Furthermore, the fetal response in acute chorioamnionitis often involves multiple chorionic vessels, is predominantly neutrophilic, and tends to radiate toward the amniotic fluid (**Fig. 12**).

MECONIUM-ASSOCIATED VASCULAR NECROSIS WITH INFLAMMATION

Meconium-associated vascular necrosis is an umbilical or chorionic fetal large vessel vasculopathy related to the toxic effects of prolonged exposure to high concentrations of meconium. This rare lesion, described in fewer than 1% of meconium-stained placentas,[52] has been associated with poor pregnancy outcome.[52,53] Histopathologic features include eosinophilic cytoplasmic degeneration and discohesion and rounding of peripheral vascular smooth muscle cells in large chorionic and umbilical vessels, associated with nuclear pyknosis (**Fig. 13**).[52] Associated neutrophils may

Fig. 12. Eosinophil-rich chorionic vasculitis. The chorionic plate vessel is infiltrated by a mixture of neutrophils and eosinophils. The inflammatory exudate radiates toward the amnion.

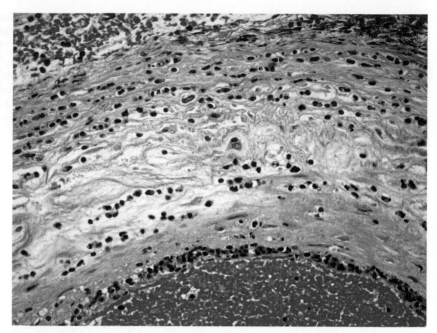

be present. Rarely, the vascular necrosis may be associated with frank umbilical cord ulceration.[52] Proposed mechanisms include meconium-induced umbilical and chorionic vasocontraction[53] as well as apoptosis of vascular smooth muscle cells.[54]

VILLITIS OF UNKNOWN ETIOLOGY WITH OBLITERATIVE FETAL VASCULOPATHY

Villitis of unknown etiology is a common lesion (5%–15% of placentas) defined by the presence of villous mononuclear cell infiltrates predominantly composed of CD8-positive maternal

Fig. 13. Meconium-associated vascular necrosis. Umbilical cord section taken from a meconium-stained placenta. Peripheral vascular smooth cells of the umbilical artery are eosinophilic, rounded, and discohesive, and have pyknotic nuclei.

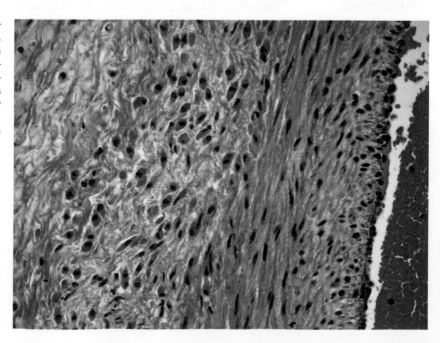

T lymphocytes.[55] The origin of this entity remains undetermined, although immune-mediated mechanisms akin to host-versus-graft rejection have been proposed. High-grade lesions have been associated with poor pregnancy outcome, including intrauterine growth restriction and recurrent reproductive loss.[55]

Chronic villitis involving the proximal stem villi may be associated with inflammation and obstructive lesions affecting the stem villous and chorionic plate fetal vessels.[55] In contrast to the acute chorionic vasculitis seen as fetal inflammatory response in the setting of acute chorioamnionitis, the obliterative fetal vasculopathy seen in association with chronic villitis is characterized by a mixed inflammatory infiltrate composed of lymphocytes and macrophages (**Fig. 14**).[55,56]

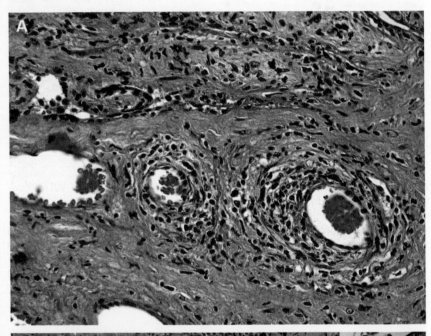

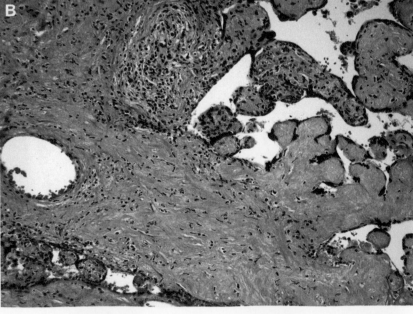

Fig. 14. Vascular involvement in chronic villitis. Stem villous vessels are infiltrated by lymphocytes and histiocytes in the setting of villitis of unknown etiology (*A*). Intense inflammation resulted in obliteration of stem villous vessels and focal avascular villi (*B*).

UMBILICAL PSEUDOVASCULITIS

Umbilical cord pseudovasculitis is a term coined to describe an autolysis-related placental artifact found in some second-trimester stillbirths.[57] The importance of this entity is that it may be mistaken for umbilical vasculitis and thus erroneously implicate ascending amniotic fluid infection in fetal demise.[57] The pseudovasculitis is manifested as numerous small, rounded degenerating cells with irregularly shaped, multilobulated nuclei within the umbilical cord vascular wall that closely resemble neutrophils (**Fig. 15A**). The changes seem restricted to the umbilical vascular smooth muscle cells and are not seen in nonumbilical vascular smooth muscle cells in fetus or placenta.[57] Useful clues alerting a pathologist to the artifactual nature of the umbilical cord pseudovasculitis include usual absence of associated chorioamnionitis, associated umbilical hypereosinophilia consistent with autolysis, associated fetal maceration and autolysis, and a regular distribution of neutrophils (in contrast to normally polarized distribution of neutrophils typical of funisitis).[57] In selected cases, ancillary studies may elucidate the true nature of the pseudoneutrophils (eg, strong staining for smooth muscle actin [see **Fig. 15B**], absent immunoreactivity for myeloperoxidase, and negative staining for chloroacetate esterase).[57]

Pitfalls
IN DIAGNOSIS UMBILICAL VASCULITIS

Umbilical pseudovasculitis

! Autolysis-related histologic artifact seen in association with postmortem fetal retention

! Small, rounded degenerating smooth muscle cells in the umbilical vessel wall with irregular, multilobed nuclei (mimicking neutrophils)

! Absence of acute chorioamnionitis (usually)

! Umbilical hypereosinophilia, consistent with autolysis

! Associated fetal maceration and autolysis

! Regular distribution of neutrophils

! Ancillary studies in equivocal cases: chloroacetate esterase, myeloperoxidase, and muscle-specific actin (rarely necessary)

ACUTE CHORIOAMNIONITIS/PLACENTAL INFLAMMATION—SPECIFIC PATTERNS

ACUTE CHORIOAMNIONITIS WITH PERIPHERAL FUNISITIS (*CANDIDA*)

Peripheral funisitis is characterized by the presence of small punctate microabscesses on the outer surface of the umbilical cord in a placenta with acute chorioamnionitis. Peripheral cord abscesses are most often seen in association with fungal infection with *Candida* sp, including *C albicans*, *C parapsilosis*, *C tropicalis*, and *C glabrata*.[58] Despite the high prevalence of vulvovaginal *Candida* colonization during pregnancy, ascending infection occurs in fewer than 1% of cases of vaginal infection and rarely causes chorioamnionitis.[59] Infrequently, *Candida* chorioamnionitis may lead to missed abortion, preterm labor, fetal death, and congenital infection[58,60–63] as well as maternal sepsis,[64] illustrating the importance of good communication between pathologists, obstetricians, and neonatologists. Foreign intrauterine bodies, such as an intrauterine device, cervical cerclage, and cervical conization, are reported risk factors.[58,61]

Grossly, lightly raised 1-mm to 2-mm yellow-white punctate plaques are disseminated on the surface of the umbilical cord (**Fig. 16A**). The remainder of the placenta usually shows membrane opacity and yellow-tan discoloration, consistent with severe acute chorioamnionitis. Microscopically, sections of umbilical cord reveal triangular-shaped microabscesses containing neutrophils and budding yeast below the amnionic lining of the cord (see **Fig. 16B**). The microabscesses, highlighted by fungal stains, may contain pseudohyphae (see **Fig. 16C**). Chorioamnionitis with marked maternal and fetal inflammatory responses is virtually always present in association with peripheral funisitis.

Although the presence of white microabscesses on the surface of umbilical cord and, less frequently, placenta, is virtually pathognomonic for *Candida* chorioamnionitis with peripheral funisitis, rare cases of peripheral funisitis caused by *Corynebacterium kutscheri*, *Haemophilus influenzae*, and *L monocytogenes* have been reported.[39] When focal and located near the placental cord insertion, peripheral funisitis is a less-specific marker for *Candida* infection and may merely represent a manifestation of conventional chorioamnionitis with extension to Wharton substance. Because of these overlapping features, the definitive diagnosis of candidal chorioamnionitis requires demonstration of fungal organisms in tissue sections.[34]

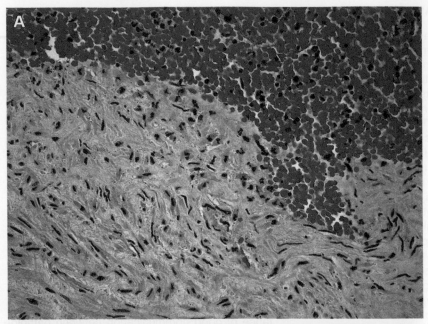

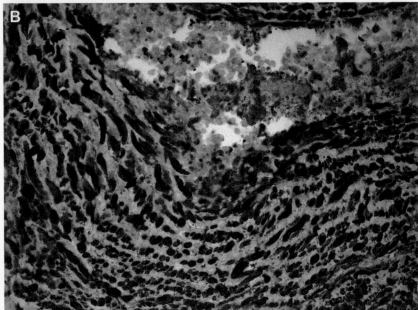

Fig. 15. Umbilical cord pseudovasculitis. Autolytic changes in umbilical vascular smooth muscle cells following fetal demise mimic neutrophils (*A*). Strong staining for smooth muscle actin demonstrates the muscle phenotype of the cells (*B*: anti-smooth muscle actin (SMA) immunohistochemistry with hematoxylin counterstain).

SUBACUTE CHORIOAMNIONITIS

Subacute chorioamnionitis is a recently defined entity characterized by a mixed inflammatory infiltrate composed of histiocytes and degenerating neutrophils in the chorionic plate.[65] Subacute chorioamnionitis has been reported in 6% of placentas from very low-birth-weight infants.[65] This condition is believed to result either from infection by organisms of low pathogenicity or from repeated bouts of mild infection in women with recurrent second-trimester and third-trimester bleeding.[39] Although increased risk for chronic lung disease has been suggested for a subgroup of very low-birth-weight infants with these placental findings, the exact clinical significance of subacute chorioamnionitis remains to be established.[65]

Fig. 16. Candida funisitis. Small, yellow-white, nodular plaques by gross examination of the umbilical cord are characteristic for *Candida* funisitis (*A*). Low-power image of the umbilical cord demonstrates triangular-shaped areas of peripheral necrosis and concentric bands of acute inflammatory exudate (*B*). Periodic acid–Schiff stain for fungus highlights pseudohyphae (*C*: periodic-acid Schiff (PAS) stain).

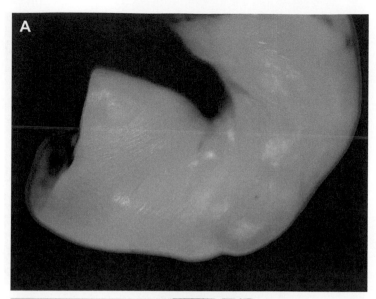

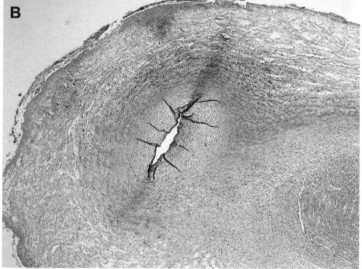

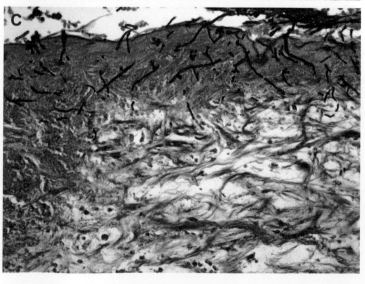

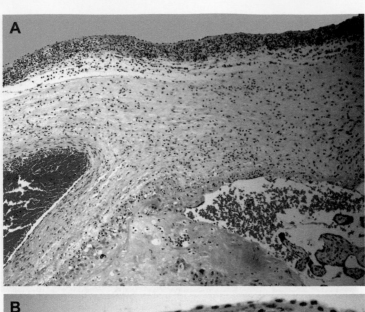

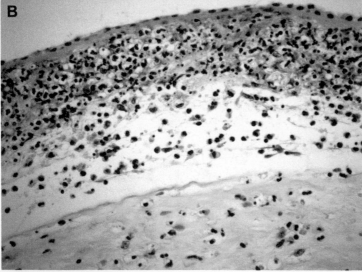

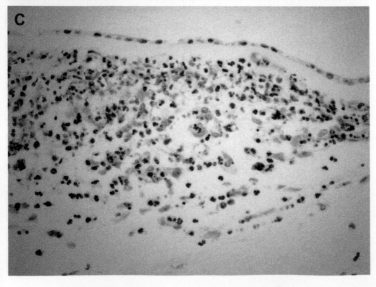

Fig. 17. Subacute chorioamnionitis. Inflammatory cell infiltration in this chorionic plate forms a continuous subamniotic band (*A*), composed of neutrophils and histiocytes (*B*). Immunostaining with CD68 highlights the histiocytic cell component (*C*: anti-CD68 immunohistochemistry with hematoxylin counterstain).

Subacute chorioamnionitis has no distinct gross appearance. Microscopically, the chorioamnion contains a mixed histiocyte-neutrophilic exudate, suggestive of prolonged duration of infection

(Fig. 17). Although in acute chorioamnionitis inflammatory cells are most prominent in subchorionic fibrin and lower chorion, the mixed inflammatory aggregates in subacute chorioamnionitis are

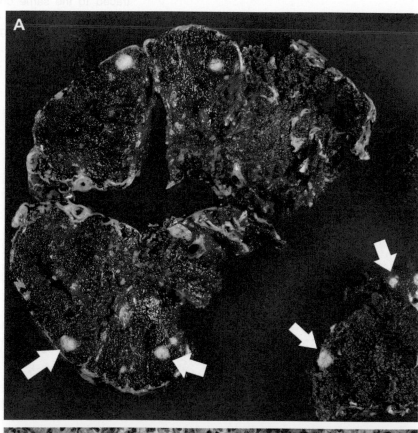

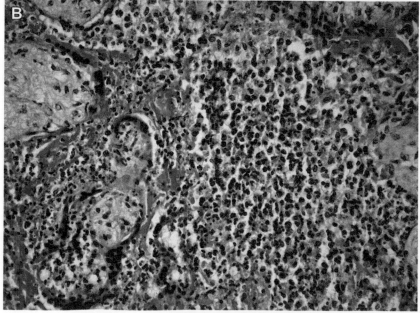

Fig. 18. Listeriosis. Multiple, firm, yellow, nodular densities (*white arrows*) are easily identifiable on the parenchymal cut sections (*A*). Microscopically, these foci correspond to intervillous abscesses (*B*). (*Courtesy of* Halit Pinar, MD, Professor of Pathology and Laboratory Medicine, Alpert Medical School of Brown University, Providence, Rhode Island.)

most numerous in the amnion and upper chorion.[34] Neutrophils may vary in number but should be present.

ACUTE INTERVILLOSITIS WITH INTERVILLOUS ABSCESSES

Neutrophilic infiltrates in the intervillous space, usually accompanied by chorioamnionitis and, in severe forms, with intervillous abscess formation, are most commonly seen with infections caused by *L monocytogenes*.[66,67] *L monocytogenes* is a gram-positive bacillus found in soil, sewage, and animal silage. The foodborne *Listeria* infections tend to occur in clusters and can often be traced to the same contaminated food source, usually dairy products or fresh produce.[68] Less common infectious agents causing the same

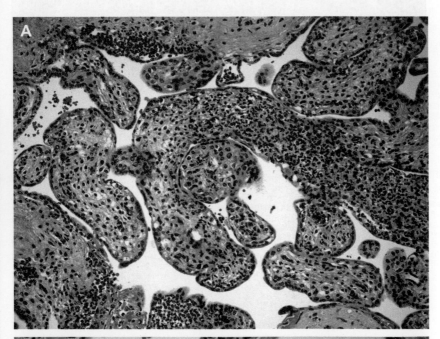

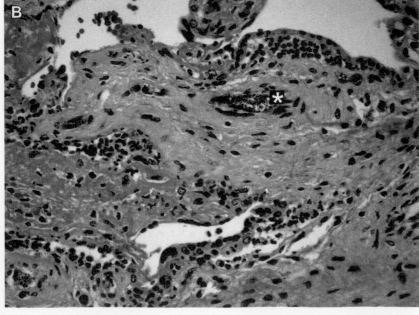

Fig. 19. Acute villitis. Acute inflammatory cell infiltration is limited to chorionic villi and involves the villous stroma (*A*). Neutrophils tend to accumulate below the trophoblast basement membrane (*B*). Intravascular bacteria (*asterisk*) are identified in stem villous vessels (*B*). Maternal blood culture was positive for group B *streptococcus*.

histologic pattern include *Campylobacter fetus*, *Chlamydia psittaci*, *Francisella tularensis*, *Klebsiella pneumoniae*, and *Coccidioides immitis*.[69–72] A recent report expanded this list of causative organisms to include 2 cases of placental *Mycobacterium tuberculosis* infection displaying acute intervillositis and villitis with intervillous abscesses, in the absence of any granulomatous reaction.[73]

In some cases, intervillous abscesses and so-called septic infarcts may be grossly visible as irregular, firm, yellow densities on the parenchymal cut surface (**Fig. 18**A). More often, the gross findings are limited to opacity and green discoloration of the membranes and pallor of the basal plate caused by associated acute deciduitis.[39] Microscopically, scattered areas of neutrophilic exudate are present within the maternal intervillous space, associated with villous necrosis and perivillous fibrin deposition (see **Fig. 18**B). Small numbers of histiocytes may be intermixed with the neutrophils. Lymphocytes, eosinophils, plasma cells, and giant cells are usually absent.[39] Infrequently, areas of acute villitis are seen in conjunction with the intervillous inflammation. In these cases, acute villitis is less extensive than the intervillositis and is presumed to reflect secondary spread to villi. Vasculitis of the stem villi may accompany the intervillous inflammation. In cases of listeriosis, gram-positive cocci are usually readily detected by tissue Gram stain.

The placental findings in cases of maternal septicemia are usually similar to those associated with listeriosis and other infections causing acute intervillositis. In maternal septicemia, perivillous fibrin deposition and villous agglutination may predominate, whereas the intervillous inflammation may be less prominent.[39,74] Causative organisms may be evident in hematoxylin-eosin–stained sections.

ACUTE VILLITIS

Acute villitis, characterized by neutrophils in fetal capillaries and stroma of distal villi with minimal intervillous component, is believed to reflect fulminant fetal sepsis. It is most often seen in association with infection by *Escherichia coli* or group B *streptococcus* and other streptococci[39] and is believed to result from hematogenous infection of the fetus followed by bacteremic spread to villi.[39]

Gross examination of the placenta affected by acute villitis may show evidence of accompanying chorioamnionitis. Acute villitis itself has no typical gross appearance. Microscopically, neutrophils are seen within villous capillaries (acute capillaritis), associated with emigration of fetal neutrophils

Placental infection: specific inflammatory patterns	
Peripheral funisitis	• *Candida* infection
Subacute chorioamnionitis	• ? Organisms of low pathogenicity
	• ? Repeated mild infection
Acute intervillositis with intervillous abscesses	• *L monocytogenes* and other bacterial infections
Acute villitis	• Maternal sepsis
	• Fetal sepsis (group B streptococcus, gram-negative bacilli)

to villous stroma (**Fig. 19**A). There is often a marked accumulation of neutrophils below the trophoblast basement membrane (see **Fig. 19**B). Bacteria may be readily evident in routine hematoxylin-eosin–stained sections (see **Fig. 19**B).

REFERENCES

1. Romero R, Espinoza J, Goncalves LF, et al. Inflammation in preterm and term labour and delivery. Semin Fetal Neonatal Med 2006;11:317–26.
2. Newton ER. Chorioamnionitis and intraamniotic infection. Clin Obstet Gynecol 1993;36:795–808.
3. Tita AT, Andrews WW. Diagnosis and management of clinical chorioamnionitis. Clin Perinatol 2010;37: 339–54.
4. Soper DE, Mayhall CG, Dalton HP. Risk factors for intraamniotic infection: a prospective epidemiologic study. Am J Obstet Gynecol 1989;161:562–6 [discussion: 566–8].
5. Gibbs RS, Duff P. Progress in pathogenesis and management of clinical intraamniotic infection. Am J Obstet Gynecol 1991;164:1317–26.
6. Yoon BH, Romero R, Moon JB, et al. Clinical significance of intra-amniotic inflammation in patients with preterm labor and intact membranes. Am J Obstet Gynecol 2001;185:1130–6.
7. Alexander JM, McIntire DM, Leveno KJ. Chorioamnionitis and the prognosis for term infants. Obstet Gynecol 1999;94:274–8.
8. Seong HS, Lee SE, Kang JH, et al. The frequency of microbial invasion of the amniotic cavity and histologic chorioamnionitis in women at term with intact membranes in the presence or absence of labor. Am J Obstet Gynecol 2008;199:375, e371–5.
9. Blume HK, Li CI, Loch CM, et al. Intrapartum fever and chorioamnionitis as risks for encephalopathy in term newborns: a case-control study. Dev Med Child Neurol 2008;50:19–24.

10. Goldenberg RL, Andrews WW, Hauth JC. Choriode-cidual infection and preterm birth. Nutr Rev 2002;60: S19–25.

11. Sperling RS, Newton E, Gibbs RS. Intraamniotic infection in low-birth-weight infants. J Infect Dis 1988;157:113–7.

12. Waites KB, Katz B, Schelonka RL. Mycoplasmas and ureaplasmas as neonatal pathogens. Clin Microbiol Rev 2005;18:757–89.

13. Silver HM. Listeriosis during pregnancy. Obstet Gynecol Surv 1998;53:737–40.

14. Roberts DJ, Celi AC, Riley LE, et al. Acute histologic chorioamnionitis at term: nearly always noninfectious. PLoS One 2012;7:e31819.

15. Hillier SL, Martius J, Krohn M, et al. A case-control study of chorioamnionic infection and histologic chorioamnionitis in prematurity. N Engl J Med 1988;319:972–8.

16. Rogers BB, Alexander JM, Head J, et al. Umbilical vein interleukin-6 levels correlate with the severity of placental inflammation and gestational age. Hum Pathol 2002;33:335–40.

17. Pacora P, Chaiworapongsa T, Maymon E, et al. Funisitis and chorionic vasculitis: the histological counterpart of the fetal inflammatory response syndrome. J Matern Fetal Neonatal Med 2002;11:18–25.

18. Yoon BH, Romero R, Park JS, et al. The relationship among inflammatory lesions of the umbilical cord (funisitis), umbilical cord plasma interleukin 6 concentration, amniotic fluid infection, and neonatal sepsis. Am J Obstet Gynecol 2000;183:1124–9.

19. Hillier SL, Witkin SS, Krohn MA, et al. The relationship of amniotic fluid cytokines and preterm delivery, amniotic fluid infection, histologic chorioamnionitis, and chorioamnion infection. Obstet Gynecol 1993; 81:941–8.

20. Kim CJ, Yoon BH, Park SS, et al. Acute funisitis of preterm but not term placentas is associated with severe fetal inflammatory response. Hum Pathol 2001;32:623–9.

21. Cherouny PH, Pankuch GA, Romero R, et al. Neutrophil attractant/activating peptide-1/interleukin-8: association with histologic chorioamnionitis, preterm delivery, and bioactive amniotic fluid leukoattractants. Am J Obstet Gynecol 1993;169:1299–303.

22. Mittal P, Romero R, Kusanovic JP, et al. CXCL6 (granulocyte chemotactic protein-2): a novel chemokine involved in the innate immune response of the amniotic cavity. Am J Reprod Immunol 2008;60: 246–57.

23. Park CW, Moon KC, Park JS, et al. The involvement of human amnion in histologic chorioamnionitis is an indicator that a fetal and an intra-amniotic inflammatory response is more likely and severe: clinical implications. Placenta 2009;30:56–61.

24. Buhimschi CS, Bhandari V, Han YW, et al. Using proteomics in perinatal and neonatal sepsis: hopes and challenges for the future. Curr Opin Infect Dis 2009; 22:235–43.

25. Leviton A, Paneth N, Reuss ML, et al. Maternal infection, fetal inflammatory response, and brain damage in very low birth weight infants. Developmental Epidemiology Network Investigators. Pediatr Res 1999;46:566–75.

26. Redline RW, O'Riordan MA. Placental lesions associated with cerebral palsy and neurologic impairment following term birth. Arch Pathol Lab Med 2000;124: 1785–91.

27. Gomez R, Romero R, Ghezzi F, et al. The fetal inflammatory response syndrome. Am J Obstet Gynecol 1998;179:194–202.

28. Thomas W, Speer CP. Chorioamnionitis: important risk factor or innocent bystander for neonatal outcome? Neonatology 2011;99:177–87.

29. Strunk T, Doherty D, Jacques A, et al. Histologic chorioamnionitis is associated with reduced risk of late-onset sepsis in preterm infants. Pediatrics 2012;129:e134–41.

30. Keenan WJ, Steichen JJ, Mahmood K, et al. Placental pathology compared with clinical outcome: a retrospective blind review. Am J Dis Child 1977;131:1224–7.

31. Redline RW, Wilson-Costello D, Borawski E, et al. The relationship between placental and other perinatal risk factors for neurologic impairment in very low birth weight children. Pediatr Res 2000;47: 721–6.

32. Redline RW. Clinically and biologically relevant patterns of placental inflammation. Pediatr Dev Pathol 2002;5:326–8.

33. Salafia CM, Weigl C, Silberman L. The prevalence and distribution of acute placental inflammation in uncomplicated term pregnancies. Obstet Gynecol 1989;73:383–9.

34. Redline RW, Faye-Petersen O, Heller D, et al. Amniotic infection syndrome: nosology and reproducibility of placental reaction patterns. Pediatr Dev Pathol 2003;6:435–48.

35. De Paepe ME, Friedman RM, Gundogan F, et al. The histologic fetoplacental inflammatory response in fatal perinatal group B-streptococcus infection. J Perinatol 2004;24:441–5.

36. Redline RW. Inflammatory response in acute chorioamnionitis. Semin Fetal Neonatal Med 2012;17: 20–5.

37. van Hoeven KH, Anyaegbunam A, Hochster H, et al. Clinical significance of increasing histologic severity of acute inflammation in the fetal membranes and umbilical cord. Pediatr Pathol Lab Med 1996;16: 731–44.

38. Kim CJ, Yoon BH, Romero R, et al. Umbilical arteritis and phlebitis mark different stages of the fetal inflammatory response. Am J Obstet Gynecol 2001;185:496–500.

39. Kraus FT, Redline RW, Gersell DJ, et al. Inflammation and infection. Placental pathology. In: Kraus FT, Redline RW, Gersell DJ, et al, editors. Washington, DC: American Registry of Pathology; 2004. p. 75–115.

40. Matoso A, Shapiro S, De Paepe ME, et al. Placental intravascular organisms: a case report. J Perinatol 2010;30:688–90.

41. Altshuler G, Hyde S. Clinicopathologic considerations of fusobacteria chorioamnionitis. Acta Obstet Gynecol Scand 1988;67:513–7.

42. Han YW, Fardini Y, Chen C, et al. Term stillbirth caused by oral Fusobacterium nucleatum. Obstet Gynecol 2010;115:442–5.

43. Gersell DJ, Phillips NJ, Beckerman K. Chronic chorioamnionitis: a clinicopathologic study of 17 cases. Int J Gynecol Pathol 1991;10:217–29.

44. Gersell DJ. Chronic villitis, chronic chorioamnionitis, and maternal floor infarction. Semin Diagn Pathol 1993;10:251–66.

45. Jacques SM, Qureshi F. Chronic chorioamnionitis: a clinicopathologic and immunohistochemical study. Hum Pathol 1998;29:1457–61.

46. Kim CJ, Romero R, Kusanovic JP, et al. The frequency, clinical significance, and pathological features of chronic chorioamnionitis: a lesion associated with spontaneous preterm birth. Mod Pathol 2010;23:1000–11.

47. Ogge G, Romero R, Lee DC, et al. Chronic chorioamnionitis displays distinct alterations of the amniotic fluid proteome. J Pathol 2011;223:553–65.

48. Stanek J, Al-Ahmadie HA. Laminar necrosis of placental membranes: a histologic sign of uteroplacental hypoxia. Pediatr Dev Pathol 2005;8:34–42.

49. Salafia CM, Ghidini A, Minior VK. Uterine allergy: a cause of preterm birth? Obstet Gynecol 1996;88:451–4.

50. Fraser RB, Wright JR Jr. Eosinophilic/T-cell chorionic vasculitis. Pediatr Dev Pathol 2002;5:350–5.

51. Jacques SM, Qureshi F, Kim CJ, et al. Eosinophilic/T-cell chorionic vasculitis: a clinicopathologic and immunohistochemical study of 51 cases. Pediatr Dev Pathol 2011;14:198–205.

52. Altshuler G, Arizawa M, Molnar-Nadasdy G. Meconium-induced umbilical cord vascular necrosis and ulceration: a potential link between the placenta and poor pregnancy outcome. Obstet Gynecol 1992;79:760–6.

53. Altshuler G, Hyde S. Meconium-induced vasocontraction: a potential cause of cerebral and other fetal hypoperfusion and of poor pregnancy outcome. J Child Neurol 1989;4:137–42.

54. King EL, Redline RW, Smith SD, et al. Myocytes of chorionic vessels from placentas with meconium-associated vascular necrosis exhibit apoptotic markers. Hum Pathol 2004;35:412–7.

55. Redline RW. Villitis of unknown etiology: noninfectious chronic villitis in the placenta. Hum Pathol 2007;38:1439–46.

56. Redline RW, Ariel I, Baergen RN, et al. Fetal vascular obstructive lesions: nosology and reproducibility of placental reaction patterns. Pediatr Dev Pathol 2004;7:443–52.

57. Genest DR, Granter S, Pinkus GS. Umbilical cord 'pseudo-vasculitis' following second trimester fetal death: a clinicopathological and immunohistochemical study of 13 cases. Histopathology 1997;30:563–9.

58. Qureshi F, Jacques SM, Bendon RW, et al. Candida funisitis: a clinicopathologic study of 32 cases. Pediatr Dev Pathol 1998;1:118–24.

59. Cotch MF, Hillier SL, Gibbs RS, et al. Epidemiology and outcomes associated with moderate to heavy Candida colonization during pregnancy. Vaginal Infections and Prematurity Study Group. Am J Obstet Gynecol 1998;178:374–80.

60. Friebe-Hoffmann U, Bender DP, Sims CJ, et al. Candida albicans chorioamnionitis associated with preterm labor and sudden intrauterine demise of one twin. A case report. J Reprod Med 2000;45:354–6.

61. Roque H, Abdelhak Y, Young BK. Intra amniotic candidiasis. Case report and meta-analysis of 54 cases. J Perinat Med 1999;27:253–62.

62. Horn LC, Nenoff P, Ziegert M, et al. Missed abortion complicated by Candida infection in a woman with rested IUD. Arch Gynecol Obstet 2001;264:215–7.

63. Diana A, Epiney M, Ecoffey M, et al. "White dots on the placenta and red dots on the baby": congenital cutaneous candidiasis—a rare disease of the neonate. Acta Paediatr 2004;93:996–9.

64. Barth T, Broscheit J, Bussen S, et al. Maternal sepsis and intrauterine fetal death resulting from Candida tropicalis chorioamnionitis in a woman with a retained intrauterine contraceptive device. Acta Obstet Gynecol Scand 2002;81:981–2.

65. Ohyama M, Itani Y, Yamanaka M, et al. Re-evaluation of chorioamnionitis and funisitis with a special reference to subacute chorioamnionitis. Hum Pathol 2002;33:183–90.

66. Driscoll SG, Gorbach A, Feldman D. Congenital listeriosis: diagnosis from placental studies. Oncologia 1962;20:216–20.

67. Vawter GF. Perinatal listeriosis. Perspect Pediatr Pathol 1981;6:153–66.

68. Southwick FS, Purich DL. Intracellular pathogenesis of listeriosis. N Engl J Med 1996;334:770–6.

69. Altshuler G, Russell P. The human placental villitides: a review of chronic intrauterine infection. Curr Top Pathol 1975;60:64–112.

70. Hyde SR, Benirschke K. Gestational psittacosis: case report and literature review. Mod Pathol 1997; 10:602–7.

71. Janssen MJ, van de Wetering K, Arabin B. Sepsis due to gestational psittacosis: a multidisciplinary approach within a perinatological center—review of reported cases. Int J Fertil Womens Med 2006;51: 17–20.

72. Sheikh SS, Amr SS, Lage JM. Acute placental infection due to Klebsiella pneumoniae: report of a unique case. Infect Dis Obstet Gynecol 2005; 13:49–52.

73. Abramowsky CR, Gutman J, Hilinski J. Mycobacterium tuberculosis infection of the placenta: a study of the early (innate) inflammatory response in two cases. Pediatr Dev Pathol 2012;15(2):132–6.

74. Bendon RW, Bornstein S, Faye-Petersen OM. Two fetal deaths associated with maternal sepsis and with thrombosis of the intervillous space of the placenta. Placenta 1998;19:385–9.

Umbilical Cord Pathology

Rebecca N. Baergen, MD

KEYWORDS

• Umbilical cord • Perinatal pathology • Stillbirth • Growth restriction

ABSTRACT

Problems and abnormalities of the umbilical cord play a significant role in perinatal morbidity and mortality. Because the umbilical cord is the lifeline of the fetus, any disruption of blood flow through the umbilical vessels can lead to severe fetal consequences.

OVERVIEW

Problems and abnormalities of the umbilical cord play a significant role in perinatal morbidity and mortality. Because the umbilical cord is the lifeline of the fetus, any disruption of blood flow through the umbilical vessels can lead to severe fetal consequences.[1-5] Mechanical obstruction of blood flow through the umbilical cord may occur secondary to compression of umbilical vessels from the fetus itself, as in cord entanglements or prolapse, by compression of susceptible membranous vessels, or by an abnormal anatomic configuration, such as true knot, abnormal coiling, abnormal length, or constriction. Often these abnormalities are seen together. For example, entanglements and knots are often seen in long cords, and excessive coiling is frequently present in cases of cord constrictions. These conditions are present for weeks or months before delivery and, therefore, can cause chronic, intermittent obstruction of blood flow, with decreased venous return of oxygenated blood from the placenta to the fetus and resultant thrombosis in the fetal circulation. If obstruction is complete, fetal death may be the eventual result.[1,2,5-9] Alternatively, more acute compression may result when a knot or entanglement tightens during descent down the birth canal and there is loss of the cushioning effect of the amniotic fluid after membrane rupture. Acute compression more often leads to fetal distress, death, or neurologic injury. Lesser degrees of obstruction can lead to poor growth or varying degrees of neurologic injury. Finally, disruption of fetal or umbilical vessels results in varying degrees of acute fetal hemorrhage, which, if severe, can result in exsanguinations and death.

The umbilical cord is normally twisted in a counterclockwise or "left" direction, with one complete spiral for approximately 5 cm of cord. The average cord length at term is approximately 55 cm, and cords less than 35 cm are considered short and those greater in 70 to 80 cm are considered long.[10-12] Cord diameter at term varies between approximately 1.2 to 1.7 cm. The cord most commonly inserts onto the placental surface in a central, paracentral or eccentric manner but may insert at the margin or into the membranes, a velamentous insertion. The cord contains two arteries and a vein within Wharton's jelly, covered by a layer of amnionic epithelium, which is contiguous with the fetal skin. Wharton's jelly is consists primarily of water, which prevents compression of umbilical vessels, but also contains ground substance and occasional macrophages and myofibroblasts. Abnormalities include (**Box 1**):

- Discoloration
- Excessive or decreased length
- Overcoiling and undercoiling
- Constrictions
- True knots
- Cord entanglements
- Velamentous insertion and/or velamentous vessels
- Single umbilical artery (SUA) or supernumerary vessels
- Thrombosis
- Hematoma and cord rupture
- Embryonic remnants
- Meconium-associated myonecrosis
- Hemangiomas.

Department of Pathology and Laboratory Medicine, New York Presbyterian Hospital, Weill Cornell Medical Center, Surgical Pathology, Starr 1002, 520 East 70th Street, New York, NY 10065, USA
E-mail address: rbaergen@med.cornell.edu

Surgical Pathology 6 (2013) 61–85
http://dx.doi.org/10.1016/j.path.2012.11.003
1875-9181/13/$ – see front matter

Box 1
Key Points: Gross Examination and Pathology

- Evaluate color
  - Normal pearly white
  - Green or brown meconium staining
    - Additional sections suggested to evaluate for possible myonecrosis
  - Yellow
    - Maternal hyperbilirubinemia
    - Possible acute funisitis—ascending infection
    - Circumscribed lesions—*Candida* infection
  - Red
    - Focal red discoloration may be due to necrosis, thrombosis or may be iatrogenic
    - Diffuse red discoloration usually due to hemolysis seen commonly in fetal demise
- Measure total of all cord fragments for length and diameter
  - Excessively long cord >70 cm
  - Excessively short cord <35 cm if all segments present
- Coiling
  - Right or left
  - Hypercoiling or hypocoiling
  - Focal constrictions
- True knots
  - Document whether tight or loose
  - Document if there is congestion of either side of knot
  - Photograph if there is a history of poor outcome or low Apgar scores
  - Untie knot and document whether it stays curled—implies chronicity
  - Additional sections through knot after untying
- Cord insertion
  - Velamentous
  - Marginal with velamentous vessels
  - Furcate, interpositional
- Number of vessels
  - SUA
  - Supernumerary vessel
- Note other abnormalities, such as thrombosis, hemorrhage, or rupture

---

GROSS LESIONS AND FEATURES

CORD DISCOLORATION

The normal cord is pearly white but may show variety of discolorations identifiable on gross examination (see **Box 1**). This is usually associated with a similar discoloration of the fetal surface and fetal membranes. Green or yellow-green discoloration is most commonly associated with meconium discharge before birth (**Fig. 1**). Brown discoloration is usually due to hemosiderin deposition from old hemorrhage (**Fig. 2**). Both of these pigments are taken up by macrophages, which are usually visible within the membranes but more difficult to identify in microscopic sections of the cord due to a general paucity of cells. Red to brown discoloration is mostly commonly

Fig. 1. Deeply meconium-stained umbilical cord with typical green to brown discoloration.

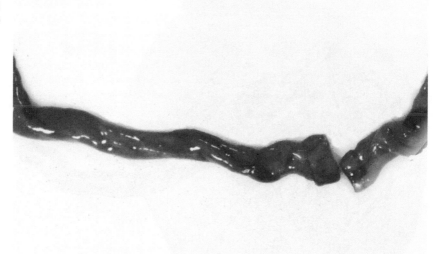

associated with hemolysis after fetal death (**Fig. 3**). Yellow discoloration is uncommon but may be present in maternal bilirubinemia (**Fig. 4**) and rarely from acute funisitis and usually only when it is necrotizing. In that case, the inflammatory cells form rings around the umbilical vessels, the cells undergo necrosis, and the necrotic debris calcifies. This leads to the presence of chalky white rings around the vessels visible on cut section (**Fig. 5**).[4,13] (Acute funisitis is discussed in more detail in the article by Gundogan and De Paepe elsewhere in this issue.) In addition, focal plaque-like discolorations of the umbilical cord may also occur in infection with *Candida* (**Fig. 6**).[4,14] Microscopically, these lesions are composed of focal collections of acute inflammatory cells, necrotic debris, and fungal organisms, which can be identified on special stains (**Fig. 7**).

UMBILICAL CORD LENGTH

Excessively long cords are estimated to occur in 4% to 6% of placentas whereas abnormally short cords have an incidence of approximately 1% to 2%.[3,14] The distinction between absolute and functional lengths is important, because a cord

Fig. 2. Fetal surface of a placenta with brown discoloration (cord is not shown in this photograph) due to hemorrhage. Histologic sections confirmed the presence of Prussian blue–positive hemosiderin-laden macrophages.

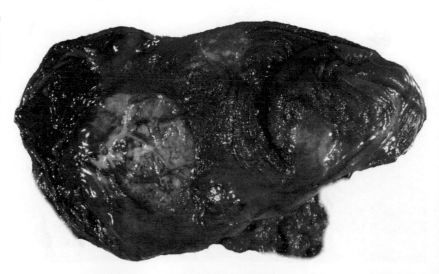

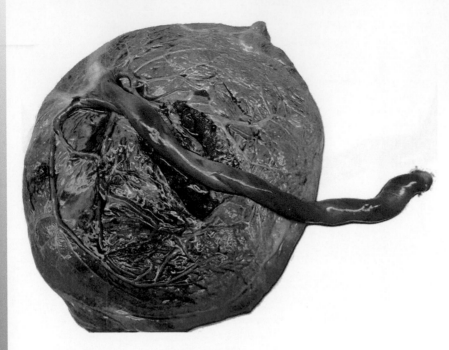

Fig. 3. Placenta and cord from a case of fetal demise. Note the reddish discoloration of the cord and fetal surface secondary to hemolysis.

that is long but entangled around the fetus is functionally short. Additionally, with respect to diagnosis of a short cord, the entire cord is almost never submitted to pathology. Up to 7 cm is left attached to the infant at delivery, and other fragments are discarded or used for blood gas determinations or other testing.[14] Thus, the length of cord submitted to pathology represents only the minimum length of the cord, not the true length, and, therefore, the diagnosis of an excessively short cord must be made with caution, if at all. For these reasons, the only accurate recording of cord length must be done at the time of delivery. Unfortunately, attempts to convince delivering physicians of the importance of this enterprise have generally failed.

Cord length seems to be determined by several factors, including gestational age, genetics, and

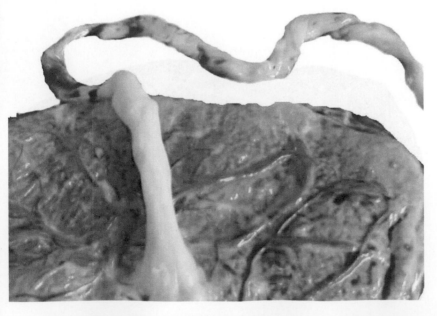

Fig.   4. Yellow-stained cord and fetal surface from a case of maternal hyperbilirubinemia.

Fig. 5. Cross-section of a cord with necrotizing funisitis. Note the white rings that partially encircle the vessels (most prominent peripherally). (*Courtesy of* Cynthia Kaplan, M.D., Stony Brook NY; with permission).

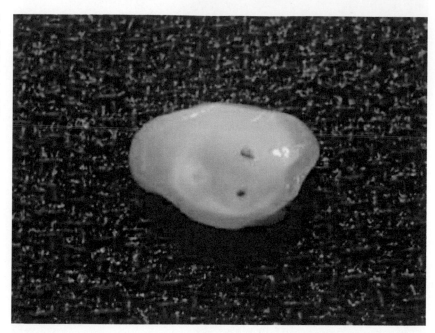

fetal movement in utero. Most of a cord's length is achieved by the 28th week of pregnancy and, although growth slows after this time, it never ceases entirely. Genetics also seems to play a role in that long cords have a tendency to recur, because mothers who deliver babies with a long cord have approximately twice the chance of a long cord in a subsequent pregnancy.[3] Longer cords are seen in male and larger babies. Movement in utero has been shown to affect cord length. Short cords are more common in situations in which there is decreased fetal movement due to congenital anomalies, such as skeletal dysplasias or trisomy 21, and where there is intrauterine constraint, such as with uterine anomalies, ectopic pregnancies, amnionic bands, and multiple gestations. Animal studies have confirmed this association.[3,4,10,14–18] This association with fetal movement is also seen in cord coiling (discussed later) where fetal activity in utero correlates with the degree of coiling.

Presumably, due to the excessive length, long cords have increased resistance to blood flow, resulting in decreased venous return, thus are associated with villous capillary congestion and thrombosis in the fetal circulation (**Fig. 8**). Long cords are also associated with other pathologic changes indicative of decreased oxygenation, including increased nucleated red blood cells and chorangiosis.[3] Long cords are also associated with an increased incidence of cord entanglement, cord prolapse, true knots, excessive coiling, and constriction.[3,4] Clinical sequelae of long cords, include fetal distress, intrauterine growth restriction, fetal demise, neonatal coagulation disorders, cerebral degenerative change, and abnormal long-term neurologic outcome.[3,4,11,14,18]

Excessively short cords are also correlated with neonatal problems, including fetal distress, low Apgar scores, depressed IQ, and developmental anomalies, in particular abdominal wall defects. Because cord length is correlated with fetal activity in utero, the essential question is whether the length of the cord is determined by prenatal central nervous system problems leading to lack of movement or whether the central nervous system problems result from perinatal problems attending the delivery of a short cord.[18] Many subsequent neonatal problems associated with short cords are related to excess traction during delivery and these include premature separation of the placenta (abruptio), cord hemorrhage, cord hematoma, cord rupture, uterine inversion, failure of descent, and prolongation of the second stage of labor.

UMBILICAL CORD COILING, TORSION, AND STRICTURE

The umbilical cord is usually coiled or twisted, mostly in a counterclockwise direction, a left twist, in a ratio of approximately 4:1.[4] Coiling is established early in gestation and has been seen by sonography as early as the 9th week. The coiling

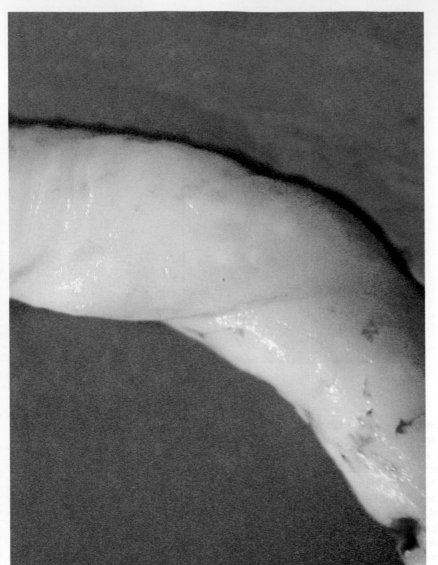

Fig. 6. Umbilical cord with infection with *Candida albicans*. Note the subtle yellow, round discolorations on the surface representing foci of necrosis.

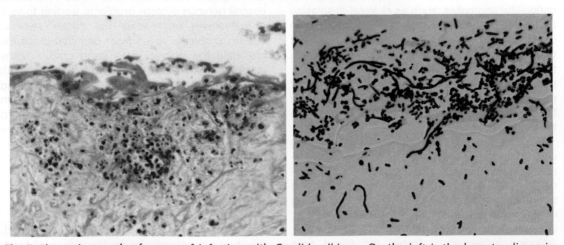

Fig. 7. Photomicrograph of a case of infection with *Candida albicans*. On the left is the hematoxylin-eosin–stained section showing mostly necrotic debris on the surface of the cord. Organisms cannot be readily identified. On the right is a Gomori methenamine silver stain of the same section clearly showing yeast forms and pseudo-hyphae (original magnification ×200).

Fig. 8. Term placenta with excessively long cord measuring more than 100 cm in length. The cord is also excessively twisted/coiled.

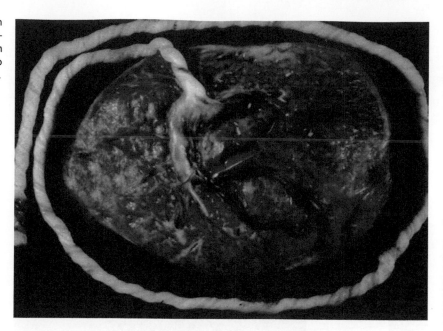

index has been used to evaluate the degree of twisting, defined as the number of coils divided by length of cord, with an average coiling index of 0.21/cm or 1 complete spiral for approximately 5 cm of cord.[2,17] Hypocoiled cords are seen in approximately 7.5% of cords; noncoiled cords are present in 4% to 5%; and hypercoiled cords are reported to be present in anywhere from 10% to 20%.[17] Similarly to cord length, coiling is believed related to fetal activity.[3,4,7,10,11,15,18]

The degree of coiling tends to be somewhat uniform throughout the length of the umbilical cord (see **Box 1**). Excessive coiling, however, may be localized and form a stricture or constriction (**Figs. 9** and **10**), often found at the fetal end of the cord and an important cause of fetal demise.[2,17,19–22] Although constriction may occur in part because of a gradually diminishing amount of Wharton jelly near the abdominal surface, it is not an artifact, as some investigators have

Fig. 9. Early fetal demise with excessively coiled cord and a constriction at the umbilicus. This is undoubtedly the cause of death.

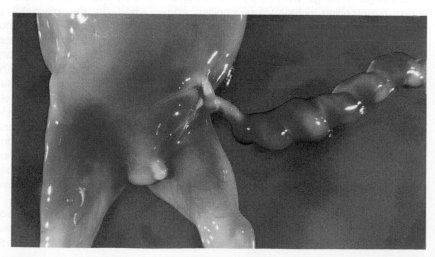

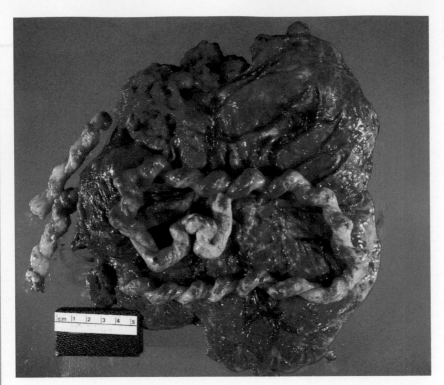

Fig. 10. Term placenta with excessively coiled cord.

suggested, and the pathologic changes associated with strictures support this, specifically the common finding of congestion on one side of the constriction and thrombosis in fetal vessels. The latter findings are proof, at least in those cases, that this is not an artifact. Constrictions are also associated with fetal growth restriction and fetal intolerance to labor.[2,4,22,23] Cord strictures are most commonly seen in hypercoiled cords and rarely seen in hypocoiled or normally coiled cords.

Pathologic findings associated with stricture and/or hypercoiling include villous capillary congestion, compression, and/or distension of the umbilical vein, long-standing degeneration of the umbilical vessels, and thrombi in the umbilical or chorionic plate vessels. Because these fetuses are often macerated and coagulation is inadequately developed in embryos, the demonstration of thrombi may be difficult in early gestation.

Hypercoiling is associated with an increase in preterm labor, low umbilical arterial pH, chronic fetal hypoxia, perinatal mortality, intrauterine growth restriction, and fetal distress.[2,7,19–23] Hypocoiling is associated with reduced fetal movement in utero and thus has been seen with increased frequency in central nervous system anomalies and previous intrauterine neurologic injury. It is also associated with fetal distress, fetal anomalies, chromosomal errors, and increased perinatal mortality.[7–9,15,22,23]

UMBILICAL CORD KNOTS

True knots of the umbilical cord occur with a frequency of 0.3% to 2.1%[9] with a higher frequency in long or hypercoiled cords.[10,17,20] They may be loose or tight (**Fig. 11**) and complex entanglements can occur. Tight knots obviously may cause compression of Wharton jelly, congestion on the placental side of the knot, and a tendency of the unknotted cord to curl if the knot has been present for a period of time (see **Box 1**). In clinically significant knots, the venous stasis that occurs often results in marked distension of the chorionic plate vessels and thrombosis of chorionic plate vessels or even the umbilical vein in some cases. False knots should not be called knots at all because they are actually local redundancies of the umbilical vessels, usually the vein (**Fig. 12**). Although some may appear complex, their nature becomes clear on careful gross inspection. At present, no clinical sequelae have been described.

True knots are more frequent with long and hypercoiled cords, multigravidas, and male fetuses.[12,17,20] Entanglement between the 2 umbilical cords of

Fig. 11. Tight true knot of the umbilical cord without real congestion on either side of the knot. In this instance there was to untoward outcome.

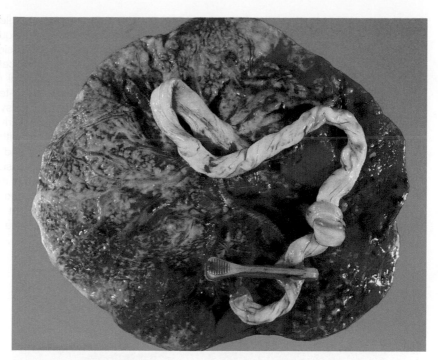

monoamnionic twins is also common. Knots are believed to develop early in gestation, weeks or months before term, when the fetus has the space to become entangled. Demise due to knots can occur at any time during gestation and has been reported even in the first trimester. Knots often do not become tight, however, until late in pregnancy when the fetus descends into the pelvis or after the onset of labor when fetal descent into the birth canal increases traction on the cord. Knots may then result in significant hypoxia and have been associated with an increased incidence of fetal distress, neurologic damage, or fetal death.[4,24] Fortunately, most true knots are not associated with adverse outcome and the overall mortality rate is approximately 10%.[4]

Fig. 12. False knot of the umbilical cord. Some false knots can be complex, like this one. They occur due to redundancies of 1 umbilical vessel, usually the vein, that develop for unknown reasons. They have no clinical consequences.

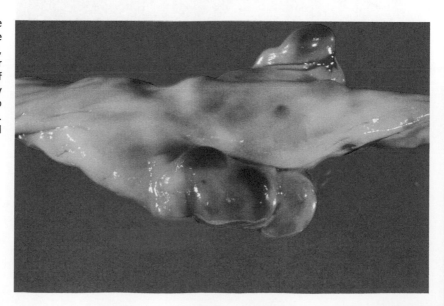

CORD ENTANGLEMENT AND CORD PROLAPSE

Entanglement of the umbilical cord can occur around any fetal part but nuchal cords are most common with an incidence of 20% at term.[3,4] Nuchal cords with 2 loops around the neck occur in 2.5% of births and 3 nuchal loops in 0.5% of births but up to 8 loops have been reported.[4] Nuchal cords have been identified as early as 10 weeks' gestation, although some of these may resolve before delivery.[25] A cord that encircles the neck in a locked pattern is of greater significance to outcome than those with an unlocked pattern.[26] Cord entanglements of any kind are more common with long cords.[3,27]

Although most entanglements are loose and have no adverse consequences, they are associated with more admissions to a neonatal ICU, a higher incidence of cesarean section delivery, low Apgar scores, fetal growth restriction, neonatal anemia, poor long-term neurologic outcome, spastic cerebral palsy, and fetal demise (**Fig. 13**).[9,24,28–31] Similarly to true knots, entanglements can tighten with fetal movement and descent during labor and delivery. If the entanglement is tight, compression of the umbilical vein can occur because it is more distensible than the arteries, resulting in decreased venous return of oxygenated blood from the placenta.[30] In some cases, this is so severe that significant anemia,

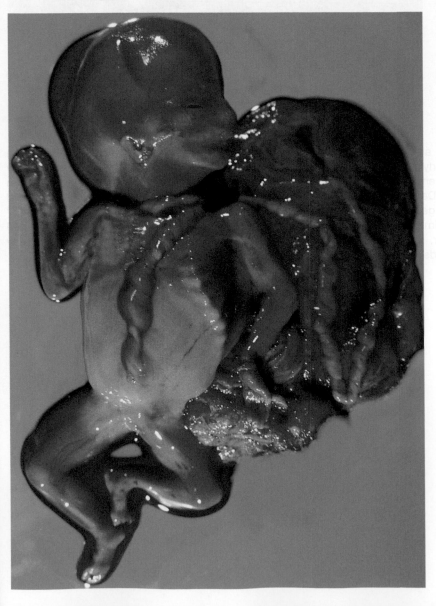

Fig. 13. Early fetal demise due to cord entanglement. Note the tight nuchal cord, which encircles the neck in a locked pattern. The cord is also excessively long and excessively coiled, conditions that commonly accompany cord entanglements.

hypovolemia, and even shock can occur.[29] Long-standing compression of the cord in entanglements can lead to thrombosis of umbilical vessels but is more commonly associated with thrombosis of the chorionic vessels.

Cord prolapse occurs when the umbilical cord precedes the fetal presenting part, which enables significant compression of cord, particularly against the cervix, during delivery. Prolapse is uncommon and is estimated to occur in 0.41% of deliveries. It is increased in multiparity, preterm labor, multiple gestation, malpresentation, low birth weight, obstetric manipulation, polyhydramnios, abruption, plavental previa, long cords, and artificial rupture of membranes with high presenting fetal parts.[3,19,32] Prolapsed cords may have serious neurologic consequences and are associated with a perinatal mortality of approximately 10% to 13%.[4] Pathologic findings are only those of acute congestion and possibly localized damage to the umbilical cord at the site of the compression, but the latter finding is rare.

CORD INSERTION

The umbilical cord normally inserts on the placental surface, more often near or at the center than elsewhere. In approximately 7% of term placentas, it has a marginal insertion in which it inserts at the edge of the placenta, and in approximately 1%, the cord inserts into the membranes, a velamentous or membranous insertion (Fig. 14).[4,14] Velamentous cord insertion is more common with twins and higher multiples and in association with a SUA. As a result of the loss of Wharton jelly as the velamentous vessels course through the membranes, they are more susceptible to thrombosis, compression, disruption, and trauma (see Box 1). Membranous vessels are not confined to velamentous cord insertions but also are present in multilobate placentas and occasionally in marginal insertions and the same susceptibility applies to these velamentous vessels.

Variations of abnormal insertions also occur. In a furcate insertion, the umbilical vessels branch before the cord inserts onto the surface of the placenta (Fig. 15). In an interpositional insertion, the cord runs parallel to the placental surface or in the membranes before its vessels branch (Fig. 16). Because these conditions are not characterized by loss of Wharton jelly, neither of these conditions is associated with adverse outcome.

Thrombosis of the velamentous arteries and veins may be seen in this insertional anomaly, presumably from compression of these easily compressible vessels. Hemorrhage can arise due to rupture of the velamentous vessels (Fig. 17). Hemorrhage from ruptured velamentous vessels, although this is uncommon, occurring in approximately 1 in 50 velamentous insertions with

Fig. 14. Velamentous insertion of the umbilical cord where the cord inserts close to the placental margin but there are many velamentous vessels arching out in both directions. These are all susceptible to damage but are intact in this case.

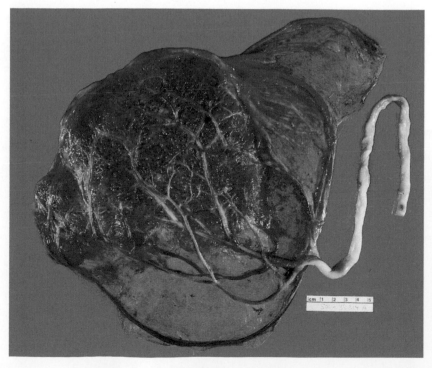

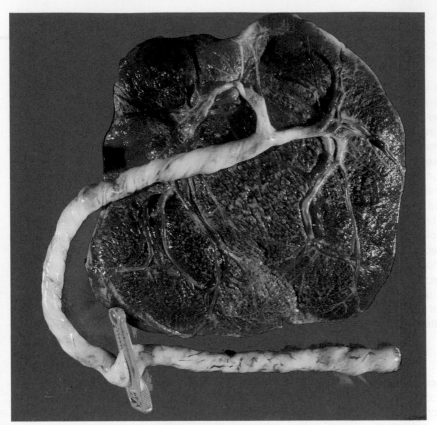

Fig. 15. Furcate insertion of the umbilical cord in which the cord divides before inserting onto the placental surface. In this case, note that the vessels are still covered by Wharton jelly and thus are protected from damage, unlike velamentous vessels.

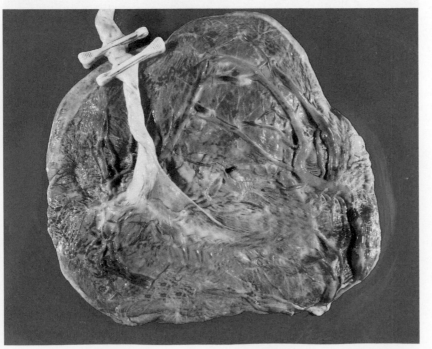

Fig. 16. This is an interpositional insertion in which the cord runs within the membranes but the vessels do not split and the cord is still protected by Wharton jelly. This is often also referred to as an amniotic web.

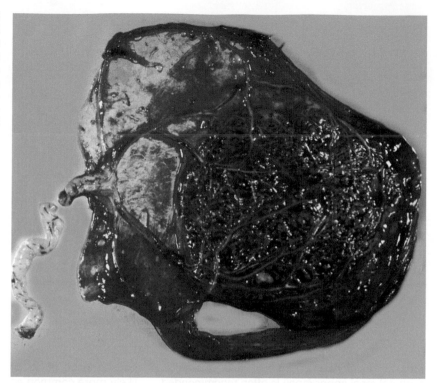

Fig. 17. Velamentous cord insertion in which a vessel has been ruptured. Note the focal hemorrhage and disruption of the vessel at the top and the hemorrhage that has dissected through the membranes. This was confirmed on histologic section.

a mortality rate estimated as high as 73%.[4,32] Abnormal fetal heart rate tracings, fetal distress, fetal growth restriction, low birth weight, low Apgar scores, neonatal thrombocytopenia, neonatal purpura, and neurologic injury have also been described.[4,27,33–35]

Examination of the placenta is essential to document the presence of velamentous vessels and to identify areas of disruption and possible hemorrhage or thrombosis. It is helpful if the possibility of a ruptured velamentous vessel is communicated to a pathologist before examination. In some cases of fetal anemia or poor outcome, the placenta should always be examined carefully for possible sources of bleeding or hemorrhage. Although hemorrhage may develop during labor and delivery due to increased forces and stress on the vessels during this time, it may commence before labor has even begun. In this case, hemosiderin-laden macrophages derived from the hemolysis of extravasated blood may be deposited around the disrupted or thrombosed vessel.

One of most serious complications of velamentous vessels is vasa previa, in which membranous vessels are present over the internal cervical os and precede the presenting fetal part. In this situation, membranous vessels may be disrupted by the exiting fetus or by an obstetric attendant who ruptures the membranes. If a vaginal delivery is attempted, the velamentous vessels are disrupted, potentially leading to fetal death due to exsanguinations or serious neurologic injury.[36,37]

SINGLE UMBILICAL ARTERY AND SUPERNUMERARY VESSELS

SUA is the most common congenital anomaly of humans (**Fig. 18**). It has an incidence of 0.5% to 1% in singletons and 8.8% in twins.[4] It can usually be detected prenatally by ultrasonography. A remnant of the second umbilical artery can sometimes be identified on microscopic examination (**Fig. 19**). Gross examination seems straightforward (see **Box 1**) but due to Hyrtl anastomoses, the 2 arteries communicate and fuse before insertion onto the surface of the placenta. In some cases, they fuse far above the cord insertion on the placenta. Therefore, documentation of an SUA should include sections from multiple areas of the cord, including segments near the fetal end.

SUA is associated with cord accidents, growth restriction, multiple gestation, maternal diabetes, antepartum hemorrhage, polyhydramnios, and oligohydramnios.[38] Congenital anomalies are present in 30% to 44.7% of infants in autopsy studies, and other placental abnormalities are found in 16.4%.[38] Renal anomalies are frequent,

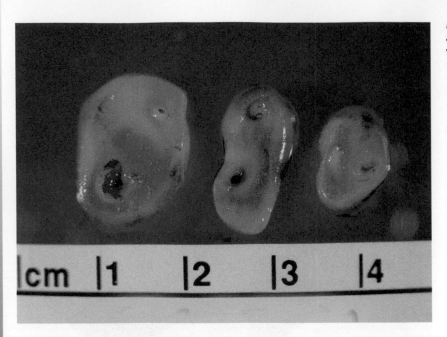

Fig. 18. Cross-sections of an umbilical cord with 2 vessels or SUA.

with an incidence of 18.5%, and, therefore, neonatal renal sonography is often recommended in cases of SUA. Intestinal atresia is also frequent in these infants. An isolated SUA, without other sonographic anomalies, does not usually affect outcome and is often found in healthy infants.

In 73% of cases, the defect locates to the left artery and associated anomalies are nearly exclusively seen with left-sided absence. Absence of 1 umbilical artery may occur as aplasia or as the

consequence of atrophy of 1 artery. Atrophy is likely more common and can sometimes be seen to have occurred on histologic examination when incomplete atrophy is present. In some cases, only a tiny muscular remnant remains. Atrophy of an artery can develop when a portion of the placenta atrophies and 1 umbilical artery loses its territory. Thus, SUA may be associated with some diminishment of placental parenchyma and is seen with increased frequncy with other

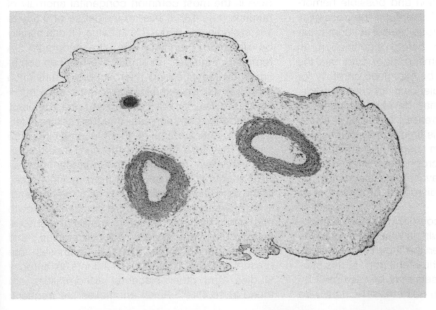

Fig. 19. Microscopic section of a cord with a SUA. Note the small residual atrophic artery at the upper left (hematoxylin-eosin, original magnification ×4).

placental shape aberrations, abnormal cord insertions, and fetal growth restriction.

More than 3 umbilical vessels is rare in humans. Normally, the right umbilical vein does not develop. Persistence of this vessel leading to a 4-vessel cord has been reported associated with congenital anomalies.[39] Occasionally, persistence of the right umbilical vein is associated with SUA Considering its rarity, when assessing the number of vessels, it is essential not to be misled by the frequent looping that occurs in many cord vessels, by false knots, or by Hyrtl anastomoses in which the umbilical arteries anastomoses before insertion onto the placental surface.

THROMBOSIS OF UMBILICAL VESSELS

Thrombosis of umbilical vessels is rare, occurring in approximately 1 in 1300 deliveries and 1 in 1000 perinatal autopsies.[23] Venous thromboses are more common than arterial thromboses, but the latter are more often lethal. Thrombi in the branches of the umbilical vessels in the chorionic plate are more common (**Fig. 20**A) but are often

Fig. 20. (*A*) Fetal surface of a placenta with a thrombus in a chorionic plate vessel. The white streak is seen within the vessel in the center of the figure. (*B*) Microscopic section of a rare calcified thrombus in an umbilical vein. The thrombus is nearly occlusive but remains partially patent. Layers of fibrin are seen on the right of figure with focal calcifications indicative of chronic obstruction to venous return (hematoxylin-eosin, original magnification ×40).

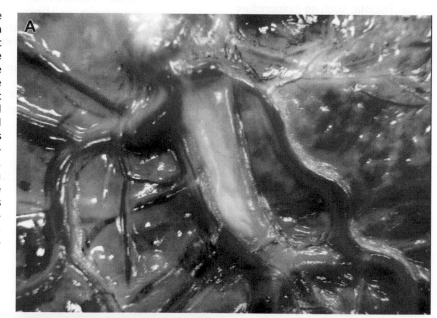

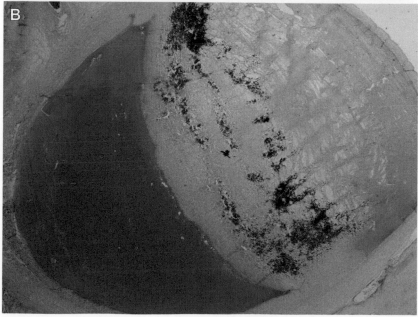

associated with the same underlying etiologies.[4] These include

- Entanglements
- Hypercoiling
- Torsion
- Knotting
- Long cords
- Velamentous insertion
- Inflammation or funisitis
- Varices
- Amnionic bands
- Maternal diabetes
- Thrombophilias of mother or infant
- Trauma, such as funipuncture

Physical compression of umbilical vessels and/or damage to vessel walls is usually the primary cause but thrombophilias, maternal diabetes, and any type of hypercoaguable state is an underlying cause. Grossly identifiable thrombi may show slight swelling and discoloration focally and may be visible on cut section (see **Boxes 2** and **3**). Microscopically, they show a typical configuration with organizing fibrin and clot within the lumen. Old thrombi may calcify and, rarely, massive calcification has made it difficult to ligate the cord at delivery (see **Fig. 20**B).

Because thrombosis can compromise the circulation, it may lead to growth restriction, fetal death, or neurologic injury.[4,23] This is particularly true of thrombosis in umbilical vessels because these are the main supply conduits of blood for the fetus. Thrombi may also break off and potentially embolize to the fetus or to the placenta, where they may cause infarction of various tissues, systemic thrombosis, or stroke.[40] Frequently, thromboses of vessels in the cord are associated with similar events in the villous ramifications.

HEMATOMA AND RUPTURE

Hematomas of the umbilical cord are rare but have serious consequences when they do occur

---

Box 2
Differential Diagnosis: Hemorrhage

- Iatrogenic
  - Evidence of cord clamp or needle puncture site
  - Clinical history
- Hematoma
  - True hematoma usually elongated and fusiform, not focal
  - Hemorrhage throughout cut section
  - Away from area of clampsing
- Hemangioma
  - Usually not distinguishable from hematoma grossly
  - Microscopically shows proliferation of vessels
  - May be associated with hemorrhage
- Thrombosis
  - Rare in the umbilical cord
  - Often difficult to differentiate grossly from hematoma
  - Often associated with thrombosis in chorionic plate vessels
- Velamentous vessels
  - Hemorrhage from disrupted velamentous vessels usually present within the membranes but also may extend to the cord itself
  - May be due to disruption of delicate vessels during delivery
  - Take sections and look for organization of hemorrhage
- Trauma
  - Often difficult to document with clinical history
  - Occasionally, needle mark may be identifiable

> **Box 3**
> **Key Points: Microscopic Umbilical Cord Pathology**
>
> - Embryonic remnants
>   - Omphalomesenteric duct
>   - Allantoic duct
>   - Vitelline vessels
> - Meconium-associated myonecrosis
>   - Usually in umbilical artery
>   - Peripheral muscle cells round up and become more eosinophilic and nucleus becomes pyknotic or disappears
>   - Usually associated with meconium macrophages in fetal membranes
> - Hematoma
>   - Acute or remote hemorrhage into Wharton jelly
>   - May be associated with compression of vessels
> - Hemangioma
>   - Proliferation of small vessels within Wharton jelly
>   - Usually of no clinical consequence
> - Thrombosis
>   - Rare in umbilical vessels
>   - May be acute or remote with calcifications
>   - Usually associated with thrombosis in chorionic plate vessels
>   - May have severe consequences for fetus

because they are associated with a 50% fetal mortality rate.[4] In large hematomas, sequelae develop secondary to blood loss but in smaller lesions morbidity and mortality occur due to compression of the umbilical vessels. Cord hematomas occur due to rupture of 1 or more umbilical vessels and underlying causes include[11,22,23]

- Short cords
- Disruption of velamentous vessels
- Trauma from amniocentesis or cordocentesis
- Inflammation or funisitis, in particular necrotizing funisitis
- Aneurysms or varices
- Hemangiomas
- Cord entanglement

Grossly, hematomas appear as elongated, fusiform swelling of the cord with marked dark red discoloration due and engorgement of blood (**Fig. 21**). This must not be confused with the iatrogenic cord hemorrhage secondary to cord clamping (see **Box 3**). Cut section reveals hemorrhage throughout the cord. If a rupture is acute,

there is blood in the amniotic fluid but no staining of the surface of the cord. If a rupture is subacute, there may be hemolysis of the extravasated blood leading to a red discoloration of the entire cord and fetal surfaces, most prominent in the areas of trauma. With more remote rupture and hemorrhage, hemosidern-laden macrophages may also be present along with organizing clot.

Aneurysms or varices are rare and show marked, focal thinning of the wall, usually of the umbilical vein. Neurologic injury or fetal death may occur from fetal hemorrhage or compression of the aneurysmally dilated veins.[41] The thinned vessel is predisposed to rupture and subsequent hematoma and ultimately can lead to adverse outcome.[42,43] When elastic stains are done on such cords, it has been repeatedly found that the elastic fibers of the vein are focally deficient (**Fig. 22**). Ulceration of the umbilical cord with hemorrhage has rarely been reported associated with duodenal atresia.[44] Rupture of the cord itself is rare, but when it occurs, it is most often at the site of its placental attachment, although it can occur anywhere. Spontaneous complete rupture

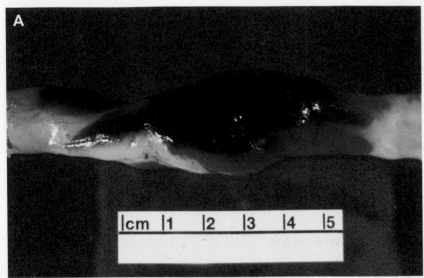

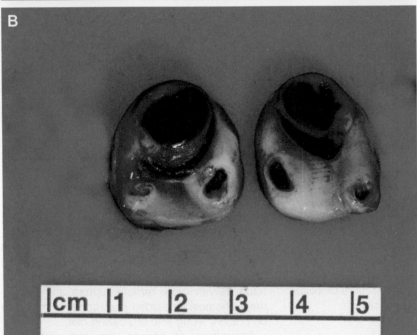

Fig. 21. (*A*) Photograph of a hematoma of the umbilical cord. Note that it has fusiform shape extending over at least 5 cm. Iatrogenic cord hemorrhage from clamping tends to be more focal. (*B*) Cut section of a cord hematoma. Note the blood within the distended vein as well as within Wharton jelly. Focal rupture of the vein was documented on histologic section.

is extremely rare[13,45–48]; most ruptures are partial and cause local hematomas or hemorrhage.

MICROSCOPIC LESIONS AND FEATURES

EMBRYONIC REMNANTS

The allantoic duct arises as a rudimentary out-pouching of the caudal portion of the yolk sac. In most cases, the duct is obliterated by 15 weeks' gestation and a remnant persists as the median umbilical ligament, connecting the umbilicus to the bladder. In approximately 15% of umbilical cords, the duct may persist.[49] They are found most frequently in the cord segments closest to the baby but may exist discontinuously throughout the cord length. They are always located between the 2 umbilical arteries and consist of flattened to

Fig. 22. (*A*) Microscopic section of an umbilical vein with marked thinning or aneurysmal dilatation—only a small thin rim of the vessel wall can be appreciated. Rupture was identified grossly and hemorrhage can be seen in the upper corner of the figure (hematoxylin-eosin, original magnification ×20). (*B*) Elastic stain of the same case as in (*A*). On the right, abundant fibers can be seen that are markedly thinned on the left side of the figure (elastic stain, original magnification ×20).

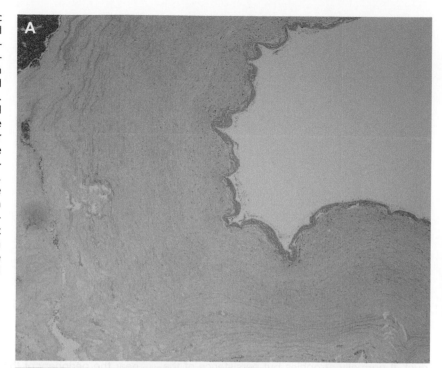

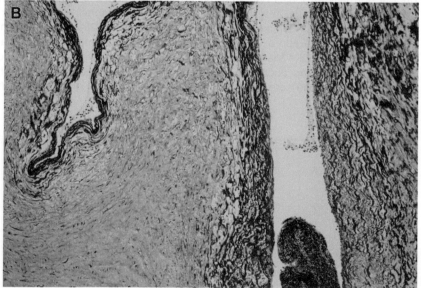

cuboidal epithelium, usually lacking a lumen. Occasionally, the epithelium is mucinous and rarely is accompanied by muscle or may calcify (**Fig. 23**). In most cases, allantoic remnants have no clinical significance but in 1 in 200,000 births[49,50] the duct is patent, connecting to the fetal bladder and, thus, may be associated with urination from the umbilical stump or development of a cyst (**Fig. 24**).[49–51]

Early in development, the midgut is connected to the yolk sac via the umbilical stalk. The connection between the gut and the yolk sac later becomes attenuated and forms the omphalomesenteric or vitelline duct. As with the allantoic

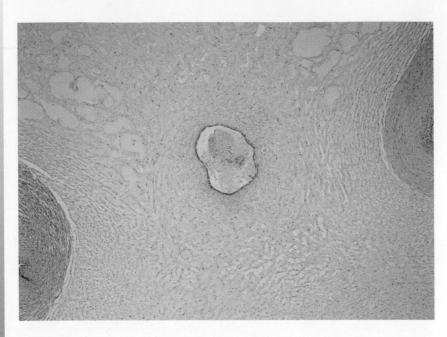

Fig. 23. Allantoic duct remnant in a typical location between the 2 umbilical arteries (hematoxylin-eosin, original magnification ×20).

duct, it normally atrophies but persistence of the duct may then be found in a approximately 1.5% of umbilical cords. Remnants of the vitelline vessels are found in approximately 7% of cords at term (Fig. 25).[49] Like allantoic ducts, remnants of omphalomesenteric ducts are more common at the fetal end of the cord but are usually found near the periphery of the cord. They are lined by columnar cells similar to intestinal epithelium (Fig. 26) and are often associated with muscle. They may occur in pairs. Being of endodermal original, this duct occasionally may contain remnants of liver, small bowel, pancreatic tissue, adrenal gland, gastric mucosa, ganglion cells, or

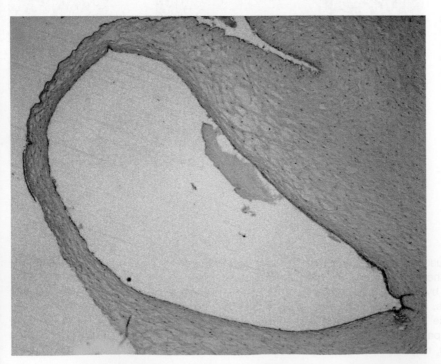

Fig. 24. Allantoic duct cyst. In this case, the cyst was not large enough to cause clinical consequences (hematoxylin-eosin, original magnification ×40).

Fig. 25. Remnants of vitelline vessels that typically form a focal area with multiple small vessels (hematoxylin-eosin, original magnification ×200).

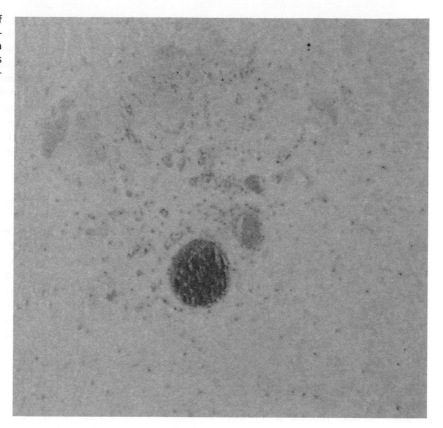

other intestinal structures.[52] Calcification or cyst formation may also occur. Remnants of omphalomesenteric ducts have uncommonly been associated with small intestinal atresia or Meckel diverticulum. Omphalomesenteric duct remnants are commonly associated with persistent vitelline vessels (see **Box 3**; **Fig. 26**).

MECONIUM-ASSOCIATED MYONECROSIS

Meconium is the intestinal content of the fetus and discharge of meconium into the amniotic fluid is a common event, particularly at term and beyond. In a small percentage of cases, meconium is aspirated by the fetus and then meconium aspiration

Fig. 26. Remnant of an omphalomesenteric duct with intestinal-type epithelium (hematoxylin-eosin, original magnification ×200).

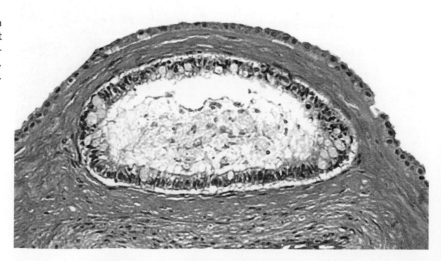

syndrome may develop, a condition associated with significant neonatal morbidity and mortality. It is often suggested, that meconium discharge is indicative of fetal distress. Although meconium discharge may be a response to fetal distress, it also frequently occurs as a physiologic event without evidence of any distress, particularly in term and post-term babies. In addition, many babies show evidence of in utero distress and in fact may die in utero without any evidence of meconium discharge. Thus, the notion that the presence of meconium is always indicative of fetal distress is unfounded.[4]

Meconium has been shown to be a noxious material, containing bile salts, cholic acid, enzymes, and other compounds.[4] Therefore, if meconium is present for a sustained period of time, it can damage the amnion, the umbilical cord, and fetal vessels. It is generally accepted that many hours of meconium exposure are required for gross staining of the umbilical cord but meconium-filled macrophages are difficult to identify in the cord because of the paucity of macrophages and because meconium pigment does not survive exposure to light.[53] After prolonged meconium exposure, damage to the umbilical cord vessels may develop, manifesting as necrosis of the vascular smooth muscle of umbilical vessels.[54] Myonecrosis most commonly involves the arteries, most likely because they are closer to the surface than the veins and carry deoxygenated blood. The muscle fibers, which are normally spindled, round up and the cytoplasm takes on a deeper eosinophilia (see **Box 3**; **Fig. 27**). The nuclei may become pyknotic and eventually disappear completely. In extreme cases, ulceration of the cord may occur.[55] In vitro studies have shown that meconium causes vasoconstriction of umbilical vessels,[54] a process that is more likely to occur with long meconium exposure and in cases of meconium-associated myonecrosis.

HEMANGIOMAS AND OTHER NEOPLASMS

Hemangiomas are benign neoplasms that may develop in the umbilical cord. They tend to occur at the placental end of the cord. Although most are small, tumors up to 18 cm in length and 14 cm in diameter and weigh up to 900 g have been reported.[56,57] They have a fairly uniform histologic appearance (**Fig. 28**), consisting of a proliferation of capillaries in loose connective tissue stroma (see **Boxes 2** and **3**). Some have more myxoma-like stroma; these are referred to as angiomyoxomas. Like chorangiomas, sequelae of hemangiomas depend on the size of the tumor and they have been associated with

- Fetal hemorrhage
- High output cardiac failure
- Elevated maternal AFP levels
- Disseminated intravascular coagulation
- Fetal hemangiomas

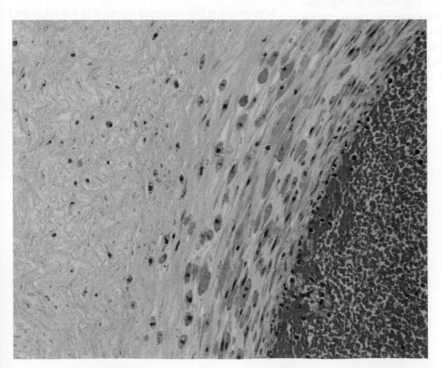

Fig. 27. Section of an umbilical artery with meconium myonecrosis. The pigmented macrophages cannot be seen in this image but the dying muscle fibers are clearly visible. The cells show increased eosinophilia and are rounded up with small, dark, pyknotic nuclei. Some fibers have completely lost their nucleus. This is the classic appearance for meconium-induced damage (hematoxylin-eosin, original magnification ×40).

Fig. 28. Hemangioma of the umbilical cord in which there is a proliferation of capillaries within the cord forming a distinct mass as opposed to vitelline vessel remnants (hematoxylin-eosin, original magnification ×200).

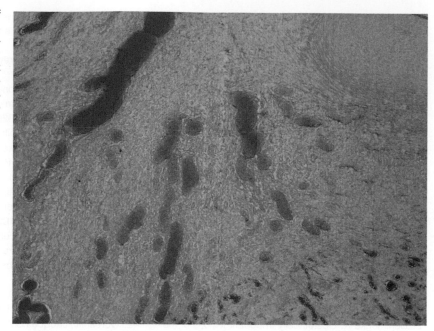

- Fetal anomalies
- Fetal death

Teratomas are rarely reported as arising in the umbilical cord but there is some controversy about their existence and their differentiation from acardiac twins.[4] Generally speaking, however, if a lesion does not contain axial skeleton or umbilical cord, it likely represents a true tumor. As with other teratomas, skin, connective tissue, and various other tissues, such as colonic or respiratory epithelium, are often present. No adverse sequelae have been reported.

REFERENCES

1. Redline RW, O'Riordan MA. Placental lesions associated with cerebral palsy and neurologic impairment following term birth. Arch Pathol Lab Med 2000; 124(12):1785–91.
2. Machin GA, Ackerman J, Gilbert-Barness E. Abnormal umbilical cord coiling is associated with adverse perinatal outcomes. Pediatr Dev Pathol 2000;3(5):462–71.
3. Baergen RN, Malicki D, Behling C, et al. Morbidity, mortality, and placental pathology in excessively long umbilical cords: retrospective study. Pediatr Dev Pathol 2001;4(2):144–53.
4. Benirschke K, et al. Pathology of the human placenta. New York: Springer Science+Business Media, Inc; 2006.
5. Grafe MR. The correlation of prenatal brain damage with placental pathology. J Neuropathol Exp Neurol 1994;53(4):407–15.
6. Redline RW. Clinical and pathological umbilical cord abnormalities in fetal thrombotic vasculopathy. Hum Pathol 2004;35(12):1494–8.
7. Peng HQ, et al. Umbilical cord stricture and overcoiling are common causes of fetal demise. Pediatr Dev Pathol 2006;9(1):14–9.
8. Murphy DJ, MacKenzie IZ. The mortality and morbidity associated with umbilical cord prolapse. Br J Obstet Gynaecol 1995;102(10):826–30.
9. Spellacy WN, Gravem H, Fisch RO. The umbilical cord complications of true knots, nuchal coils, and cords around the body. Report from the collaborative study of cerebral palsy. Am J Obstet Gynecol 1966;94(8):1136–42.
10. Miller ME, Higginbottom M, Smith DW. Short umbilical cord: its origin and relevance. Pediatrics 1981; 67(5):618–21.
11. Naeye RL. Umbilical cord length: clinical significance. J Pediatr 1985;107(2):278–81.
12. Rayburn WF, Beynen A, Brinkman DL. Umbilical cord length and intrapartum complications. Obstet Gynecol 1981;57(4):450–2.
13. Chasen ST, Baergen RN. Necrotizing funisitis with intrapartum umbilical cord rupture. J Perinatol 1999; 19(4):325–6.
14. Baergen RN. Manual of Benirschke and Kaufmann's pathology of the human placenta. New York: Springer; 2005.

15. Miller ME, Jones MC, Smith DW. Tension: the basis of umbilical cord growth. J Pediatr 1982;101(5):844.

16. Moessinger AC, et al. Umbilical cord length as an index of fetal activity: experimental study and clinical implications. Pediatr Res 1982;16(2):109–12.

17. Boue DR, Stanley C, Baergen RN. Placental pathology casebook. Long umbilical cord with torsion and diffuse chorionic surface vein thrombosis: multiple associated congenital abnormalities including destructive encephalopathy. J Perinatol 1995;15(5):429–31.

18. Snider W. Placental casebook. J Perinatol 1997;17(4):327–9.

19. de Laat MW, et al. Hypercoiling of the umbilical cord and placental maturation defect: associated pathology? Pediatr Dev Pathol 2007;10(4):293–9.

20. de Laat MW, et al. The umbilical coiling index in complicated pregnancy. Eur J Obstet Gynecol Reprod Biol 2007;130(1):66–72.

21. Strong TH Jr, Elliott JP, Radin TG. Non-coiled umbilical blood vessels: a new marker for the fetus at risk. Obstet Gynecol 1993;81(3):409–11.

22. Benirschke K. Obstetrically important lesions of the umbilical cord. J Reprod Med 1994;39(4):262–72.

23. Heifetz SA. Thrombosis of the umbilical cord: analysis of 52 cases and literature review. Pediatr Pathol 1988;8(1):37–54.

24. Hershkovitz R, et al. Risk factors associated with true knots of the umbilical cord. Eur J Obstet Gynecol Reprod Biol 2001;98(1):36–9.

25. Collins JH, et al. Nuchal cords: timing of prenatal diagnosis and duration. Am J Obstet Gynecol 1995;173(3 Pt 1):768.

26. Collins JH. Umbilical cord accidents: human studies. Semin Perinatol 2002;26(1):79–82.

27. Earn AA. The effect of congenital abnormalities of the umbilical cord and placenta on the newborn and mother; a survey of 5,676 consecutive deliveries. J Obstet Gynaecol Br Emp 1951;58(3):456–9.

28. Sornes T. Umbilical cord encirclements and fetal growth restriction. Obstet Gynecol 1995;86(5):725–8.

29. Vanhaesebrouck P, et al. Tight nuchal cord and neonatal hypovolaemic shock. Arch Dis Child 1987;62(12):1276–7.

30. Shepherd AJ, Richardson CJ, Brown JP. Nuchal cord as a cause of neonatal anemia. Am J Dis Child 1985;139(1):71–3.

31. Gambhir PS, et al. Chronic umbilical cord entanglements causing intrauterine fetal demise in the second trimester. Pediatr Dev Pathol 2011;14(3):252–4.

32. Lin MG. Umbilical cord prolapse. Obstet Gynecol Surv 2006;61(4):269–77.

33. Baergen RN, Benirschke K. Manual of pathology of the human placenta. New York: Springer; 2011.

34. Heinonen S, et al. Perinatal diagnostic evaluation of velamentous umbilical cord insertion: clinical, Doppler, and ultrasonic findings. Obstet Gynecol 1996;87(1):112–7.

35. Shanklin DR. The influence of placental lesions on the newborn infant. Pediatr Clin North Am 1970;17(1):25–42.

36. Torrey WE Jr. Vasa previa. Am J Obstet Gynecol 1952;63(1):146–52.

37. Cordero DR, et al. A non-hemorrhagic manifestation of vasa previa: a clinicopathologic case report. Obstet Gynecol 1993;82(4 Pt 2 Suppl):698–700.

38. Heifetz SA. Single umbilical artery. A statistical analysis of 237 autopsy cases and review of the literature. Perspect Pediatr Pathol 1984;8(4):345–78.

39. Puvabanditsin S, et al. Four-vessel umbilical cord associated with multiple congenital anomalies: a case report and literature review. Fetal Pediatr Pathol 2011;30(2):98–105.

40. Kraus FT, Acheen VI. Fetal thrombotic vasculopathy in the placenta: cerebral thrombi and infarcts, coagulopathies, and cerebral palsy. Hum Pathol 1999;30(7):759–69.

41. Fortune DW, Ostor AG. Umbilical artery aneurysm. Am J Obstet Gynecol 1978;131(3):339–40.

42. Qureshi F, Jacques SM. Marked segmental thinning of the umbilical cord vessels. Arch Pathol Lab Med 1994;118(8):826–30.

43. Schreier R, Brown S. Hematoma of the umbilical cord. Report of a case. Obstet Gynecol 1962;20:798–800.

44. Bendon RW, et al. Umbilical cord ulceration and intestinal atresia: a new association? Am J Obstet Gynecol 1991;164(2):582–6.

45. Walker C, Ward J. Intrapartum umbilical cord rupture. Obstet Gynecol 2009;113(2 Pt 2):552–4.

46. Naidu M, et al. Umbilical cord rupture: a case report and review of literature. Int J Fertil Womens Med 2007;52(2–3):107–10.

47. Garland JM. Undiagnosed spontaneous rupture of umbilical cord. Clin Med (Northfield II) 1963;70:785–6.

48. Garland JM. Undiagnosed spontaneous rupture of the umbilical cord. Can Med Assoc J 1961;85:376.

49. Jauniaux E, et al. Embryonic remnants of the umbilical cord: morphologic and clinical aspects. Hum Pathol 1989;20(5):458–62.

50. Schaefer IM, et al. Giant umbilical cord edema caused by retrograde micturition through an open patent urachus. Pediatr Dev Pathol 2010;13(5):404–7.

51. Zangen R, et al. Umbilical cord cysts in the second and third trimesters: significance and prenatal approach. Ultrasound Obstet Gynecol 2010;36(3):296–301.

52. Lara-Diaz VJ, et al. Ectopic liver within the umbilical cord in a very preterm infant from a multiple gestation. Pediatr Dev Pathol 2011;14(5):422–5.

53. Morhaime JL, et al. Disappearance of meconium pigment in placental specimens on exposure to light. Arch Pathol Lab Med 2003;127(6):711–4.

54. Altshuler G, Hyde S. Meconium-induced vasocon-traction: a potential cause of cerebral and other fetal hypoperfusion and of poor pregnancy outcome. J Child Neurol 1989;4(2):137–42.

55. Labarrere C, et al. Absence of Wharton's jelly around the umbilical arteries: an unusual cause of perinatal mortality. Placenta 1985;6(6):555–9.

56. Vougiouklakis T, et al. Ruptured hemangioma of the umbilical cord and intrauterine fetal death, with review data. Pathol Res Pract 2006;202(7): 537–40.

57. Heifetz SA, Rueda-Pedraza ME. Hemangiomas of the umbilical cord. Pediatr Pathol 1983;1(4): 385–98.

Fetal Thrombotic Vasculopathy
Perinatal Stroke, Growth Restriction, and Other Sequelae

Frederick T. Kraus, MD

KEYWORDS

• Fetal thrombotic vasculopathy • Clots • Placental oxygen • Fetal circulation

ABSTRACT

Clots in the fetal circulation of the placenta may occlude or narrow the lumens of fetal vessels sufficiently to diminish the placental oxygen and nutritional exchange, causing significant reduction in placental function. When extensive, growth restriction, neonatal encephalopathy, and stillbirth may occur. Propagation of clots in other organs, such as brain, kidney, and liver, may affect the function of these organs, resulting in infarcts and neonatal stroke. This article presents an account of the placental pathology and clinical sequelae of this condition, called fetal thrombotic vasculopathy.

OVERVIEW

Fetal thrombotic vasculopathy (FTV) is a vascular thrombotic condition causing obstruction of arteries and veins in the fetal circulation of the placenta, resulting in ischemic changes in the villi peripheral to the obstruction. When sufficiently extensive, FTV may cause a reduction in functional placental reserve or in other cases may be associated with additional thrombotic or thromboembolic events in the somatic vessels of the fetus itself. When extensive, the former condition can lead to fetal growth restriction or stillbirth, whereas the latter may result in infarcts of various fetal structures, such as the brain, kidney, or, rarely, an extremity, such as an arm or leg. As with intravascular clotting in general, causal factors of FTV include a combination of the triad of stasis (by compression of cord or aberrant vessels); a thrombophilic state, both genetic (eg, protein S or factor V Leiden) and acquired (anticardiolipin antibody

Key Features
FTV: POTENTIAL MORPHOLOGIC OR CLINICAL ASSOCIATIONS AND SEQUELAE

Obstructive cord lesion or cord accident (common)

Admit to neonatal ICU; normal at discharge (common)

Neonatal encephalopathy (%)

Cerebral palsy (rare); includes cerebral infarct, porencephalic cyst, hypoxic-ischemic encephalopathy

Stillbirth (uncommon)

Intrauterine growth restriction (uncommon)

Oligohydramnios

Maternal diabetes mellitus (common)

Maternal autoimmune disease (lupus, anticardiolipin antibodies, and so forth) (uncommon)

Severe acute respiratory syndrome (rare)

Cytomegalovirus, *Toxoplasma gondii* (rare)

Transverse limb reduction (rare)

Maternal thrombophilic state (occurs equally in nonthrombophilic mothers)

and so forth); and vascular injury (inflammatory and localized compression). The most serious outcomes include growth restriction, neurologic injury, and perinatal death.

PREVALENCE

In an unselected series of 1153 deliveries, FTV was identified histologically in 11 placentas (1%),

Department of Obstetrics and Gynecology, Washington University School of Medicine, Campus Box 8064, 4566 Scott Avenue, St Louis, MO 63110, USA
E-mail address: krausf@wudosis.wustl.edu

Surgical Pathology 6 (2013) 87–100
http://dx.doi.org/10.1016/j.path.2012.10.001
1875-9181/13/$ – see front matter © 2013 Elsevier Inc. All rights reserved.

including 1 case of maternal gestational diabetes and 2 newborns small for gestational age; the remaining 9 mothers and newborns were clinically normal.[1] In a selected series of 2910 placentas submitted for clinical indications from a total of 19674 deliveries, 183 placentas (6%) had histologic FTV.[2]

CLINICAL FEATURES

Before delivery, FTV is clinically silent, with no predelivery warning of its presence. As discussed previously, FTV occurs more frequently in placentas selected for clinical study than in unselected pregnancies, but the factors involved in selection of placentas for pathologic study are diverse and nonspecific: maternal hypertension and diabetes mellitus, fetal growth restriction, abnormal fetal heart rate during labor, and so forth. Ultrasound and other imaging techniques do not detect FTV. When there seems to be some sort of fetal distress during labor, there is no way to suggest that the actual cause of these symptoms is FTV until the placenta is examined. In most cases, when FTV is identified on placental examination, the newborn usually appears well, there are no subsequent clinical abnormalities in the nursery, and the newborn goes home on schedule. Especially in more extensive or severe cases, FTV is associated significantly with neonatal encephalopathy,[3] cerebral palsy,[4] intrauterine growth restriction,[5] stillbirth, oligohydramnios, and fetal cardiac anomalies.[6] Cerebral infarcts may be the most common specific cerebral lesion associated with placental FTV.[7]

Other fetal structural anomalies attributed to vascular disruption (including thrombi) include porencephaly, cerebral infarcts, bowel atresias, gastroschisis, unilateral renal absence, cleft lip or palate, and transverse limb or digit reduction.[8]

RISK FACTORS

The most significant predisposing abnormalities are problems resulting in vascular stasis. These include cord prolapse, hypercoiling, and velamentous insertion.[9,10] Large vessel thrombi have a similar effect. FTV is a major finding in cases of stillbirth, even after the vascular features secondary to stillbirth itself are excluded.[6] In a study of 130 stillbirths in Australia, proved perinatal cytomegalic inclusion infection occurred in 20 cases; FTV was found disproportionately in more (60%) of the cytomegalovirus cases compared with a smaller number (28%) of the noninfected cases. FTV may occur more

---

Box 1
Risk factors for fetal thrombotic vasculopathy

Stasis: cord compression and cord hypercoiling

Maternal diabetes mellitus

Neonatal encephalopathy

Growth restriction

Stillbirth

---

frequently in association with maternal diabetes mellitus.[1] Extensive FTV was discovered in the placentas of 2 women convalescent in the third trimester with severe acute respiratory syndrome during an outbreak in Hong Kong[11]; the 2 newborns were growth restricted.

The possibility of a correlation between placental FTV and parental or fetal thrombophilias has been suggested by anecdotal observations and some earlier studies.[12–15] Later observations, controlled by comparing FTV cases with non-FTV cases, found similar proportions of maternal thrombophilias in the FTV and non-FTV cases.[16–18] FTV and thrombophilias occur together, but a thrombophilia alone does not seem to increase the prevalence of FTV.

Box 1 summarizes risk factors for FTV.

GROSS FEATURES

Thrombi in the larger vessels of the chorionic plate are often visible on gross examination (**Fig. 1**). Distension of the chorionic plate vessels (**Fig. 2**) should prompt a search for thrombosed fetal vessels and for devascularized villi by selecting multiple tissue blocks for histologic confirmation. Regions to select for this purpose include pale triangular regions with a base at the maternal surface (**Fig. 3**). Areas of villous parenchyma peripheral to an occluded vein are often darker red and congested. Older lesions may become firm and depigmented, eventually with a gray-white color. Even large lesions can often be indistinct and difficult to recognize. Formalin fixation may accentuate the appearance of lesions that were not apparent on sectioning of the fresh placenta.

FTV is commonly associated with functionally significant or potentially obstructive lesions of the umbilical cord, including velamentous insertion, hypercoiling, abnormally long cord, and effects of compression and stasis, such as fetal vascular ectasia and major fetal vessel thrombosis.[9,19]

Box 2 summarizes the gross morphology of FTV.

Fig. 1. A recent thrombus caused expansion of a large fetal artery in the chorionic plate, near the cord insertion, at the left margin.

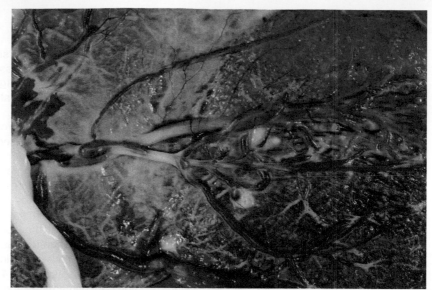

Fig. 2. Note the distended vessels in the chorionic plate, as seen in cross-sections of the placenta. Extensive FTV was present in all 12 microscopic sections from widely distributed areas, resulting in dilatation and congestion of vessels proximal to zones of obstruction. (*From* Kraus FT, Redline RW, Gersell DJ, et al. Placental Pathology. Washington, DC: American registry of Pathology; 2004:144; with permission.)

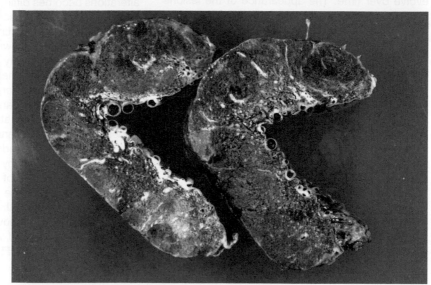

Fig. 3. Multiple areas of FTV form pale triangular areas with base at the maternal surface. This newborn had severe neonatal encephalopathy. Avascular villi from this placenta are shown in Fig. 10.

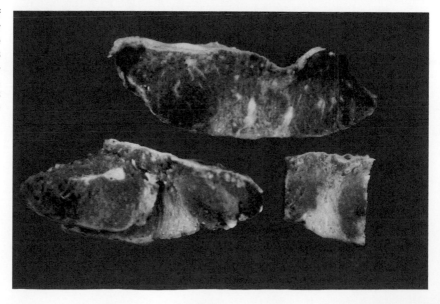

MICROSCOPIC FEATURES

The microscopic patterns of the vascular lesions grouped under the general term, *fetal thrombotic vasculopathy*, vary, especially as the lesions evolve over time. The appearance of the lesions in the larger vessels of the chorionic plate and stem vessels differs from that of the lesions in the capillaries of the terminal villi.

Thrombi in larger vessels have an evolving sequence similar to the histologic changes in thrombosed veins and arteries in adults. Acutely, the vessel wall is distended; the clot becomes adherent as the endothelial cells lyse and disappear and often develops a layered appearance with strata of red cells alternating with leukocytes and fibrin (**Fig. 4**). The breakdown of the endothelial interface allows red blood cells to extravasate and become distributed in variable numbers into the vessel wall (**Fig. 5**).

A variant early lesion is a focal accumulation of fibrin, with or without edema, beneath the vascular endothelium of stem vessels, called *fibrinous vasculosis*.[20] In some cases, stem vessels become narrowed by expanded subendothelial organizing masses of connective tissue matrix, lesions called *intimal fibrin cushions* (**Fig. 6**).[21] Focal calcification in these lesions is generally accepted as evidence of increasing chronicity.

Progressively, as thrombi age and become chronic, spindle cells resembling fibroblasts appear within the thrombus, forming a pattern called *septation*, in which the fragmenting red cells are divided into multilocular spaces (**Fig. 7**). Eventually the vessel lumen becomes obliterated, so that only an indistinct outline remains; red blood cells, distorted and fragmented, may persist even in the lumen and in the degenerated vascular wall (**Fig. 8**). Calcification may occur focally in the vessel wall as well as in the clot itself (see **Figs. 4** and **6**). Histologic distinction between arteries and veins after these chronic alterations becomes difficult or impossible.

Hemorrhagic endovasculopathy (HEV) is a vasodisruptive process affecting fetal vessels, from the larger stem vessels down to fetal capillaries. At early stages, the integrity of the vessel wall is lost and fragmented endothelial nuclei persist, intermixed with masses of erythrocytes that spill out into the villous stroma and dissect into the walls of larger vessels. The stem vessel wall in HEV appears consistently disrupted with extravasation of red cells. The affected villi in HEV may appear filled, even expanded, by stromal hemorrhage. In time, the stem vessels of both FTV and HEV may show septation and the villi eventually become avascular and hyalinized.

I have been able to show that villi in the distribution of a large placental vein showed the hemorrhagic pattern of HEV (**Fig. 9A**),[2] suggesting that

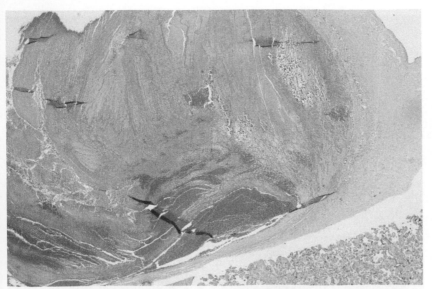

Fig. 4. Layered blood elements formed progressively over a period of several days in this thrombus occluding a large chorionic plate vessel. Note more recent stratification of red blood cells alternating with layers of fibrin and leukocytes at bottom left. There is an older pale blue granular zone of calcification near the right margin (hematoxylin-eosin, original magnification ×15).

Fig. 5. Chorionic plate artery (*right*) occluded by thrombus several days old, with prominent infiltration by fibroblasts. Note the extravasation of red blood cells at the endothelial margin. There are clumps of fibrin within the clot (hematoxylin-eosin, original magnification ×200).

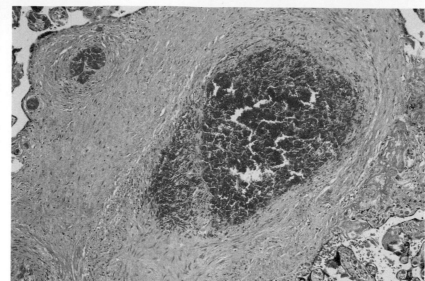

Fig. 6. This chronic intimal fibrin cushion forms an expanded mass within the wall of a large chorionic plate artery, bulging into the lumen. A more recent lesion would contain intramural fibrin or fibrinoid. An adherent mural thrombus may sometimes be present. Focal calcification, as in this image, is common (hematoxylin-eosin, original magnification ×300).

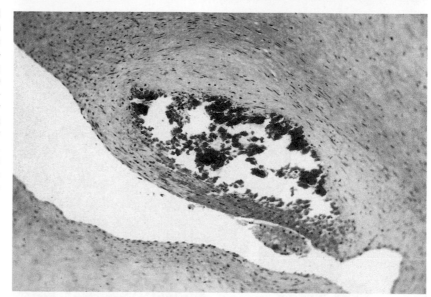

Fig. 7. Septation in a stem artery is characterized by strands of spindle-shaped fibroblastic cells that dissect into the lumen, separating clusters of red cells into small loculated spaces (hematoxylin-eosin, original magnification ×200). This is from the same placenta as shown in Figs. 4, 5, and 11. This process begins multifocally in areas of stasis in approximately 2 days and becomes extensive after 2 or more weeks. (*From* Genest DR. Estimating the time of death in stillborn fetuses: II. Histologic evaluation of the placenta; a study of 71 stillborns. Obstet Gynecol 1992; 80:585–92; with permission.)

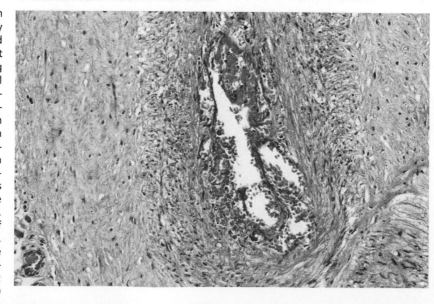

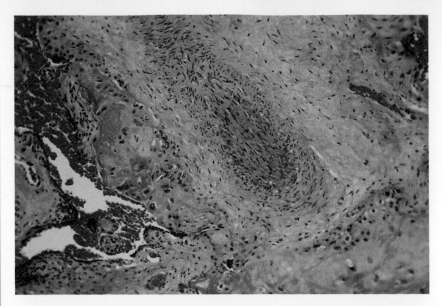

Fig. 8. This is an older occluded stem vessel, with completely obliterated lumen. Scattered degenerating red blood cells persist in the organized central area (hematoxylin-eosin, original magnification ×100).

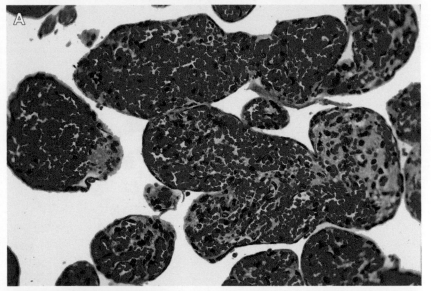

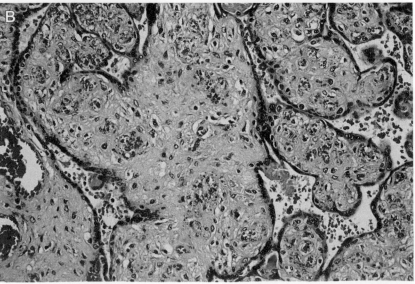

Fig. 9. (*A*) Acute villous lesion. This instance of more extensive acute intravillous hemorrhage was traced to an occlusive thrombus in a large vein just before joining the umbilical vein. (*B*) Acute villous lesion. Fetal villous capillary lesions of recent (2–4 days) duration show disappearance of most endothelial cells, extravasation, and fragmentation of red blood cells, in a region of stasis downstream from a recent stem vessel thrombus (hematoxylin-eosin, original magnification ×300).

Fig. 10. Old, chronic avascular hyalinized villi show mineralization in the basal lamina beneath the trophoblastic layer, visible in this hematoxylin-eosin–stained section. Such hyalinized villous lesions were extensive in multiple sections of this placenta (hematoxylin-eosin, original magnification ×200). This is the same same placenta as shown grossly in **Fig. 3**.

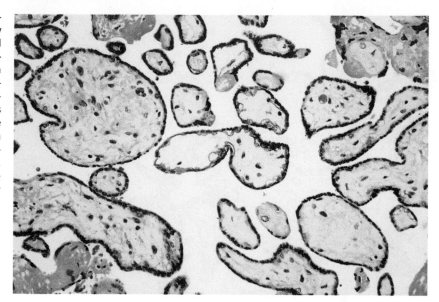

this may be a variant of FTV in which the main occlusive vessel is sometimes a large placental vein. The clinical and pathologic features of typical FTV and HEV have many similarities. The villi and villous capillaries in the regions of placenta served by the occluded veins or arteries no longer function. In recent lesions (2–5 days), the capillary endothelial cells are at first fragmented (see Fig. 9B); then the red cells, also fragmented, are extravasated, sometimes extensively into the villous stroma (see **Fig. 9**A). Ultimately, both capillaries and red cells disappear (**Fig. 10**). In chronic villous lesions (4–5 weeks), only an acellular hyalinzed core remains, surrounded by the villous trophoblast, which remains viable (**Fig. 11**). The trophoblast layer survives because it is kept alive

Fig. 11. These villi, from the same placenta as shown in Figs. **4**, **5**, and **7**, show chronic villous changes of FTV at the margin of a much larger lesion. The villi clustered at left are avascular and hyalinzed, in contrast to some adjacent normally perfused villi at right. The fetus associated with this placenta experienced intrauterine death just 36 hours before delivery. There were both old and recent thrombi in the fetal vessels, and multiple clusters of hyalinized avascular villi were present in this placenta. The intravascular clotting in-jury in this placenta began many days, possibly even weeks, before the fetal death. No symptoms were detected during the course of this carefully monitored pregnancy (hematoxylin-eosin, original magnification ×200).

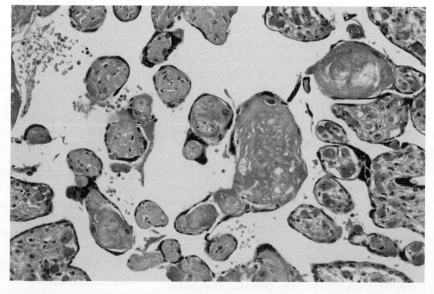

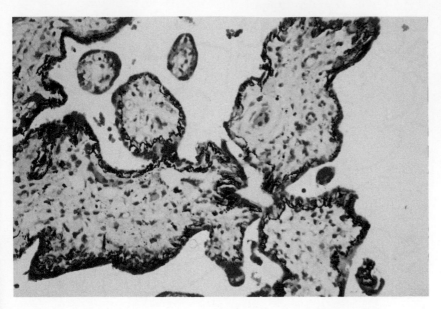

Fig. 12. Avascular hyalinized villi after Prussian blue stain for iron show dark blue linear deposits in the basement membranes beneath the trophoblast layer (Prussian blue, original magnification ×200).

by the continued circulation of maternal blood in the intervillous space. Iron is deposited in the basement membrane beneath the trophoblast (**Fig. 12**) and in small clumps in the villous stroma as the red cells disappear.

Box 3 summarizes the microscopic morphology of FTV.

Box 3
Microscopic morphology of fetal thrombotic vasculopathy

Stem vessels, chorionic plate vessels
Recent thrombi are adherent to the vessel wall, the endothelium is gone, and there is focal or extensive red cell extravasation.

Older, chronic thrombi have a fibroblastic infiltrate into the thrombus, with marked red blood cell extravasation and fragmentation; areas of fibrovascular sclerosis and endothelial cushions are often calcified.

Distal chorionic villi
In recent lesions, variably sized clusters of villi have stromal-endothelial karyorrhexis and red blood cell extravasation. The intervillous space is normal and the syncytiotrophoblastic epithelium survives.

In chronic lesions, the clusters of villi are now avascular with hyalinized stroma, but the trophoblastic cover still persists. The basal lamina beneath the trophoblast becomes mineralized (iron stain positive).

DIFFERENTIAL DIAGNOSIS

INTRAUTERINE FETAL DEATH

The histologic changes in vascular morphology after intrauterine fetal death, like the vascular changes in FTV, result from cessation of blood flow through the fetal vessels, except that the changes are diffuse throughout the entire placenta. The vascular changes are all approximately the same age, however, which depends on the length of time between fetal death and delivery. In contrast, the clusters of avascular villi of FTV form well-circumscribed clusters, surrounded by normally perfused villi. The endothelial cells fragment and the blood in larger stem vessels after fetal death is soon invaded by spindle-shaped fibroblasts, but the layered strata of leukocytes, fibrin, and red cells characteristic of thrombi in flowing blood does not occur. Red cells extravasate into the adjacent stroma. It takes approximately 2 days for the early changes of FTV to appear in villi,[22] so older, avascular hyalinzed villi or other well-established FTV changes identified within a 48-hour interval between fetal death and delivery (see **Fig. 12**) are truly pathologic FTV lesions, even though the stillborn (see **Fig. 12** description) died 36 hours before delivery.[23]

CHRONIC VILLITIS WITH OBLITERATIVE FETAL VASCULOPATHY

The larger affected areas are grossly indurated, with a gray-tan color and irregular blotchy outlines

Fig. 13. These are cross-sections of a placenta with extensive localized areas of chronic villitis. The affected areas are firm, pale, and generally well circumscribed, with functional placental villi in-between.

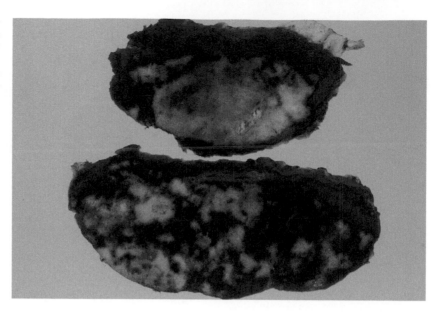

(**Fig. 13**). Stem villi involved by foci of chronic villitis may be infiltrated by the inflammatory process, and blood vessels may become thrombosed due to local endothelial injury (**Fig. 14**). The thrombi are generally limited to inflamed stem villi, but downstream avascular villi are not necessarily always involved in the inflammatory process. The inflamed villous stroma is infiltrated by predominately CD8-positive maternal T-lymphocytes and macrophages (predominately activated Hofbauer-type fetal macrophages).[24]

Groups of villli may become agglutinated by fibrin on the villous surfaces. Clusters of downstream terminal villi are avascular and hyalinized, as seen with FTV. Unlike with FTV, there is no evidence of cord occlusion.

MESENCHYMAL DYSPLASIA

The placenta is usually enlarged; chorionic plate vessels are conspicuously, even aneurysmally, dilated, tortuous, and often contain large mural

Fig. 14. Chronic villitis causing agglutination of villi at left. The occlusive stem vessel thrombus just below center resulted in downstream ischemia of clusters of avascular villi at right (hematoxylin-eosin, original magnification ×100).

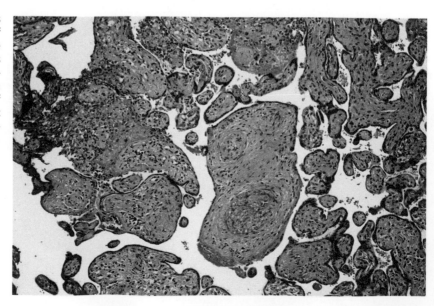

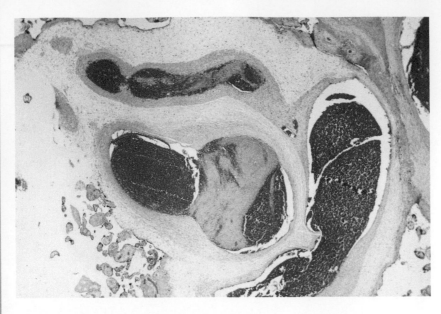

Fig.   15. Mesenchymal dysplasia. Dilated, aneurysmal stem vessels are partially occluded by thrombi and surrounded by excessive amounts of edematous mesenchyme (hematoxylin-eosin, original magnification ×15).

thrombi (**Fig. 15**). Many large, vesicular, swollen, edematous villi have an appearance suggestive of molar villi (**Fig. 16**). Placental ultrasound images are often interpreted as partial or complete hydatidiform mole. There is an increased amount of edematous mesenchymal villous stroma. Trophoblastic hyperplasia, a feature of partial or complete moles, is not present.[25] The fetus, typically female, may appear normal, but is often growth restricted, and some fetuses are stillborn, depending on the amount of functioning placenta available to the fetus. There is an association with Beckwith-Wiedemann syndrome in approximately one-third of cases.

INFARCT

The intervillous space in FTV remains open and perfused by maternal blood, whereas the intervillous space of an infarct is collapsed as the villi become adherent, separated only by thin strands of fibrin. The syncytiotrophoblast cover of infarcted villi undergoes necrosis and disappears, whereas the trophoblast surface of villi in FTV remains viable. In time, all of the cellular components of an infarct undergo necrosis and nuclear staining disappears throughout.

Table 1 presents a summary of differential diagnoses.

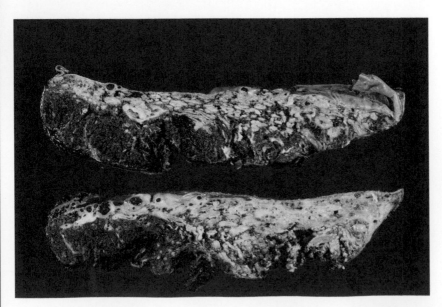

Fig. 16. Mesenchymal dysplasia. Many enlarged subchorionic villi contain abundant pale gray connective tissue; some have dilated stem vessels. A prominent component of more normal villous parenchyma at left contrasts with the markedly dysmorphic component at the right. (*Courtesy of* Deborah J. Gersell, MD, St. John's Mercy Medical Center, St Louis, MO; with permission.)

Table 1
Differential diagnosis of fetal thrombotic vasculopathy

FTV Versus	Helpful Distinguishing Features
Intrauterine fetal death	• Fetal vascular changes appear generally uniform in all placental sections
Chronic villitis	• Patchy lymphohistio-cytic infiltrate in villi • Inflammation in walls of thrombosed vessels
Mesenchymal dysplasia	• Extreme vascular distension: varicosities • Scattered large hy-dropic mesenchymal villi • Vessel proliferation

IMPACT ON OUTCOME

Placentas affected by FTV result in a 9-fold increase in prevalence of stillbirth, a 6-fold increase in cardiac abnormalities, and a 2-fold increase in growth restriction,[6] in comparison with normal placentas. The odds ratio for preterm birth is also increased.[6] Some newborns with FTV may have clinical or autopsy evidence of thrombotic lesions elsewhere in the fetal circulation. Infarcts in the brain, which may occur before birth (Fig. 17), have been demonstrated in perinatal autopsies.[2,26] In a study of 186 neonatal stroke patients in the Canadian Pediatric Ischemic Stroke Registry, only 12 had placental pathologic examinations, but of these 12, 6 had thrombi in cord, chorionic plate vessels, or other features of FTV.[27] FTV is also an important cause of hypoxic-ischemic encephalopathy, especially when associated with obstructive umbilical cord problems.[28] An autopsy study of stillbirths that correlated neuropathology with placental pathology found that FTV correlated with neuronal injury (nuclear karyorrhexis) in the brain.[29]

Instances of gangrene of an arm or leg associated with FTV are rare,[30] but dramatic, when they occur.[31] Some cases of bowel atresia have also occurred in this context, as a feature of vascular disruption (Fig. 18).[8] Placental vein thrombi appeared to have had some significance in the development of a case of twin reversed arterial perfusion sequence reported by Steffensen and colleagues.[32] In a similar context, sudden, rapid onset of twin-twin transfusion syndrome occurred as the result of a thrombus forming in one of the balancing AV anastomoses in a monochorionic twin placenta.[33]

Both fetal somatic thrombi and placental thrombi (FTV) give no specific sign or symptom of their presence until fetal death occurs or growth restriction becomes apparent. There may be reduction of amniotic fluid, but this is nonspecific, and growth restriction has many causes. FTV was one of the main placental lesions (27% of cases of

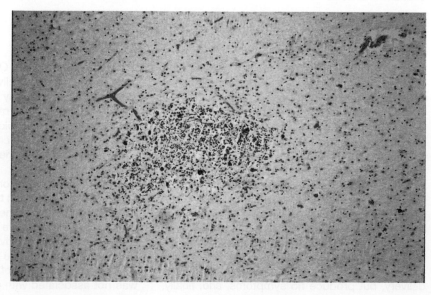

Fig. 17. This cerebral infarct has chronic histologic features, associated with thrombi in the fetal circulation in the placenta, possibly the result of embolism to the middle cerebral artery. The central necrosis, focal calcification, and marked astrocytic proliferation indicate at least several days' duration. The newborn had bradycardia during labor and severe neonatal encephalopathy but lived only 2.5 hours after birth; the placenta showed extensive chronic FTV with many clusters of avascular hyalinized villi. Both the FTV and the cerebral infarct occurred prenatally, long before the delivery (hematoxylin-eosin, original magnification × 100).

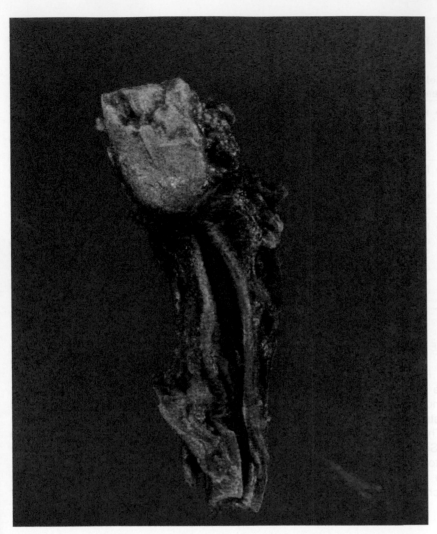

Fig. 18. Esophageal atresia associated with extensive placental FTV. Very recent fetal death in utero occurred at 32 weeks. The largest fetal vessels at the chorionic plate appeared dilated and congested. The cord had a single umbilical artery and was tightly wrapped multiple times about the left leg of the fetus, resulting in compression marks on the leg. There were several large stem vessel thrombi; both old hyalinized villi and more recent hemorrhagic villi with extravasated red blood cells were present. Instances of atresia in the digestive tract have been attributed to vascular disruptions, most likely caused by thrombi. Unfortunately, attempts to relate bowel atresia to placental pathology are not commonly made.

severe intrauterine growth restriction) causing reduced or reversed end diastolic blood flow, as demonstrated by umbilical cord blood flow Doppler velocimetry.[5]

FTV may increase progressively as the process of intravascular thrombosis extends within the placenta. Thus, FTV tends to reduce placental function progressively without causing perceptible injury until the cumulative effects of reduced placental reserve and the stress of labor onset combine to cause heart rate abnormalities, such as bradycardia, fetal distress, and even late perinatal stillbirth. It should be emphasized that FTV, as well as other pathologic processes that affect the placenta, commonly begin long before delivery, but produce no symptoms, and, finally, as injury progresses, may produce nonspecific stress related alterations, such as bradycardia,

occur at onset of labor. Often it is at this stressful time, hours before delivery, that the reduced placental function finally causes acute injury to the brain, kidneys, and other organs of the fetus, even though it is the older placental pathologic lesions that initiated the chain of events that culminated in the serious injuries that the newborn must face after delivery.

Growth restriction is common when involvement is more extensive. When the placenta is also small for gestational age, the cumulative effects of reduced size and more extensive lesions may enhance the destructive effects of reduced placental function on the organs of the fetus.

Long-term follow-up of newborns with FTV that was not associated with either reduced placental function, in the absence of symptomatic clots in the somatic circulation is not available.

UMBILICAL CORD THROMBI

Cord thrombi may be evident grossly as localized areas of fusiform enlargement or discoloration. Old thrombi may calcify. They may be associated with knots, torsion, amniotic bands, varices, infection, compression, or velamentous insertion. The umbilical vein is most commonly affected.

Thrombi in umbilical cord vessels may be partly or completely occlusive. There is a strong association with fetal morbidity, including growth restriction, and two-thirds are stillborn. Heifetz[34] found an incidence of 1:1000 perinatal autopsies, increasing to 1:250 in high-risk pregnancies. In an autopsy series of 317 consecutive stillbirths at 15 to 40 weeks gestation, Avigliano and colleagues[35] found 32 cases with thrombi in cord vessels, an incidence of 1:10. The larger incidence in this report may be related to an acceptance of fibrin identified only in phosphotungstic acid-hemotoxylin stains of cord as evidence of clots, even if lacking adherence and changes at the clot-endothelial interface in some cases; others in this study did show loss of endothelium and extravasation of red cells at the inner vessel margin. The umbilical vein was most often involved. Cord abnormalities (eg, knots and hypercoiling) were present in 13 cases. Cord thrombi and FTV do occur together, but not invariably, in this series, as well as in my experience.

REFERENCES

1. Pathak S, Lees CC, Hackett G, et al. Frequency and clinical significance of placental histological lesions in an unselected population at or near term. Virchows Arch 2011;459:565–72.
2. Kraus FT, Acheen VI. Fetal thrombotic vasculopathy in the placenta: cerebral thrombi and infarcts, coagulopathies, and cerebral palsy. Hum Pathol 1999; 30:759–69.
3. McDonald DG, Kelehan P, McMenamin JB, et al. Placental fetal thrombotic vasculopathy is associated with neonatal encephalopathy. Hum Pathol 2004;35:875–80.
4. Redline RW. Severe fetal placental vascular lesions in term infants with neurologic impairment. Am J Obstet Gynecol 2005;192:452–7.
5. Dicke JM, Huettner P, Yan S, et al. Umbilical artery Doppler indices in small for gestational age fetuses. Correlation with adverse outcomes and placental abnormalities. J Ultrasound Med 2009;28:1603–10.
6. Saleemuddin A, Tantbirojn P, Sirois K, et al. Obstetric and perinatal complications in placentas with fetal thrombotic vasculopathy. Pediatr Dev Pathol 2010; 13:459–64.
7. Takenouchi T, Kasdorf E, Engel M, et al. Changing pattern of perinatal brain injury in term infants in recent years. Pediatr Neurol 2012;46:106–10.
8. Gilbert-Barness E, Van Allen MI. Vascular disruptions. In: Gilbert-Barness E, editor. Potter's pathology of the fetus and infant. 2nd edition. St Louis (MO): Mosby; 2007. p. 176–200.
9. Redline RW. Clinical and pathological umbilical cord abnormalities in fetal thrombotic vasculopathy. Hum Pathol 2004;35:1494–8.
10. Tantbirojn P, Saleemuddin A, Sirois K. Gross abnormalities of the umbilical cord: related placental histology and clinical significance. Placenta 2009; 30:1083–8.
11. Ng WF, Wong SF, Lam A, et al. The placentas of patients with severe acute respiratory syndrome: a pathophysiological evaluation. Pathology 2006; 38:210–8.
12. Arias F, Romero R, Joist H, et al. Thrombophilia: a mechanism of disease in women with adverse pregnancy outcome and thrombotic lesions in the placenta. J Matern Fetal Med 1998;7:277–86.
13. Khong TY, Hague WM. Biparental contribution to fetal thrombophilia in discordant twin intrauterine growth restriction. Am J Obstet Gynecol 2001;185:244–5.
14. Redline RW, Pappin A. Fetal thrombotic vasculopathy: the clinical significance of extensive avascular villi. Hum Pathol 1995;26:80–5.
15. Vern TZ, Alles AJ, Kowal-Vern A, et al. Frequency of Factor V Leiden and Prothrombin G20210A in placentas and their relationship with placental lesions. Hum Pathol 2000;31:1036–43.
16. Ariel IB, Anteby E, Hamani Y, et al. Placental pathology in fetal thrombophilia. Hum Pathol 2004; 35:729–33.
17. Leistra-Leistra MJ, Timmer A, van Spronsen FJ, et al. Fetal thrombotic vasculopathy in the placenta: a thrombophilic connection between pregnancy complications and neonatal thrombosis? Trophoblast Research. Placenta 2004;25(Suppl A):S102–5.
18. Mousa HA, Alfirevic Z. Do placental lesions reflect thrombophilic state in women with adverse pregnancy outcome? Hum Reprod 2000;15:1830–3.
19. Parast MM, Crum CP, Boyd TK. Placental histological criteria for umbilical flow restriction in unexplained stillbirth. Hum Pathol 2008;39:948–53.
20. Scott JM. Fibrinous vasculosis in the human placenta. Placenta 1983;4:87–100.
21. De Sa DJ. Intimal cushions of foetal placental veins. J Pathol 1973;110:347–52.
22. Genest DR. Estimating the time of death in stillborn fetuses: II. Histologic evaluation of the placenta; a study of 71 stillborns. Obstet Gynecol 1992;80: 585–92.
23. Redline RW. Villitis of unknown etiology: noninfectious chronic villitis in the placenta. Hum Pathol 2007;38:1439–46.

24. Parveen Z, Tongson-Ignacio JE, Fraser CR, et al. Placental mesenchymal dysplasia. Arch Pathol Lab Med 2007;131:131–7.

25. Kaiser-Rogers KA, McFadden DE, Livasy CA, et al. Androgenetic/biparental mosaicism causes placental mesenchymaql dysplasia. J Med Genet 2006;43: 187–92.

26. Thorarensen O, Ryan S, Hunter J, et al. Factor V Leiden 19 mutations: an unrecognized cause of hemiplegic cerebral palsy, neonatal stroke, and placental thrombosis. Ann Neurol 1997;42:372–5.

27. Elbers J, Viero S, MacGregor D, et al. Placental pathology in neonatal stroke. Pediatrics 2011;127: e722–9.

28. Wintermark P, Boyd TK, Gregas MC, et al. Placental pathology in asphyxiated newborns meeting the criteria for therapeutic hypothermia. Am J Obstet Gynecol 2010;203(6):579.e1–9.

29. Chang KT, Keating S, Costa S, et al. Third trimester stillbirths: corrlative neuropathology and placental pathology. Pediatr Dev Pathol 2011;14:345–52.

30. Hoyme HE, Jones KL, Van Allen MI, et al. Vascular pathogenesis of transverse limb reduction defects. J Pediatr 1982;101:839–43.

31. Kraus FT, Redline RW, Gersell DJ, et al. Placental Pathology. Washington, DC: American Registry of Pathology; 2004.

32. Steffensen TS, Gilbert-Barness E, Spellacy W, et al. Placental pathology in trap sequence: clinical and pathogenetic implications. Fetal Pediatr Pathol 2008;27:13–29.

33. Nikkels PG, Van Gemert MJ, Sollie-Szarynska KM, et al. Rapid onset of severe twin-twin transfusion syndrome caused by placental venous thrombosis. Pediatr Dev Pathol 2002;5:310–4.

34. Heifetz SA. Thrombosis of the umbilical cord; analysis of 52 cases and literature review. Pediatr Pathol 1988;8:37–54.

35. Avagliano L, Marconi AM, Candiani M, et al. Thrombosis of the umbilical vessels revisited. An observational study of 317 consecutive autopsies at a single institution. Hum Pathol 2010;41:971–9.

Maternal Floor Infarction and Massive Perivillous Fibrin Deposition

Ona Marie Faye-Petersen, MD[a],*, Linda M. Ernst, MD[b]

KEYWORDS

- Maternal floor infarction • Massive perivillous fibrinoid • Placental infarction • Perivillous fibrin
- Placental fibrin • Placental ischemia

ABSTRACT

Maternal floor infarction (MFI) and massive perivillous fibrin deposition (MPVFD) are pathologically overlapping placental disorders with characteristic gross and shared light microscopic features of excessive perivillous deposition of fibrinoid material. Although rare, they are associated with high rates of fetal growth restriction, perinatal morbidity and mortality, and risks of recurrence with fetal death. The cause of the extensive fibrinoid deposition is unknown, but evidence supports involvement of maternal alloimmune or autoimmune mechanisms. This article presents an updated discussion of features, placental histopathologic differential diagnosis, possible causes, clinical correlates, and adverse outcomes of the MFI/MPVFD spectrum.

OVERVIEW

Maternal floor infarction (MFI) and massive perivillous fibrin deposition (MPVFD) are rare (incidence 0.028%–0.5% of deliveries),[1–4] closely related placental lesions of unclear etiopathogenesis but associated with high perinatal morbidity, mortality, and recurrence risks. MFI[5] refers to a lesion grossly characterized by a yellowish, thickened maternal floor, and, histologically, by extensive, basal rind-like depositions of fibrin material. Although its appearance is grossly suggestive of laminar infarction, microscopically, chorionic villi in MFI are atrophic and widely separated by cloaks of this fibrin material, instead of displaying a predominant pattern of ischemic injury (ie, villous crowding, excessive syncytial knot formation, and necrosis). Thus, the term, *infarction*, is a misnomer. Also, perivillous fibrinoid deposition often extends beyond the basal plate, variably entrapping villi and obliterating the intervillous space. Fox and Elston[6] proposed the descriptive term, *MPVFD*, to denote this constellation of features, and Katzman and Genest[7] provided useful semiquantitative diagnostic criteria. Their subclassifications enable diagnostic uniformity and more meaningful, comparative clinicopathologic and outcomes studies between MFI/MPVFD and other entities showing excessive perivillous fibrinoid deposition. As discussed in this article, the composition of the perivillous fibrin and/or fibrin-like complex (fibrinoid) is incompletely understood, and its deposition likely progresses during gestation. The terms, *MFI* and *MPVFD*, are often used interchangeably in the literature, because most investigators[5,8] consider them variants of a common pathologic spectrum. Thus, for the purposes of this discussion, *MPVFD* is used to refer to the spectrum of changes of MFI and MPVFD, and *fibrinoid* to refer to the perivillous material.

GROSS FEATURES

MPVFD typically results in a small-for-gestational date, dense (stiff) placenta with a firm, yellow-white, thickened-appearing maternal surface (**Fig. 1**). Serial sections of classic forms exhibit a yellowish basal layer or rind of fibrinoid (**Fig. 2**). More commonly, fibrinoid deposition is more diffuse, with vertically oriented, pale trabeculae

[a] The University of Alabama at Birmingham, 619 South 19th Street, Birmingham, AL 35249-7331, USA;
[b] Northwestern University, Olson 2-454, 303 East Chicago Avenue, Chicago, IL 60611, USA
* Corresponding author.
E-mail address: onafp@uab.edu

Surgical Pathology 6 (2013) 101–114
http://dx.doi.org/10.1016/j.path.2012.10.002
1875-9181/13/$ – see front matter © 2013 Elsevier Inc. All rights reserved.

Key Points
OF **MPVFD**

1. MPVFD is also known as MFI

2. MPVFD is a rare but important lesion of unknown cause but strong evidence for involvement of auto/alloimmune mechanisms in most studies; other etiologies possible

3. The Classic prenatal ultrasonographic findings are fetal intrauterine growth restriction, oligohydramnios, and dense hyperechoic placenta

4. MPVFD has a high morbidity and mortality rate, with high risks of neurologic injury and of recurrence

5. The placenta is usually small and dense with friable, granular trabeculae of fibrinoid deposition

6. The predominant histopathologic feature is basal deposition of abundant fibrinoid with variable upwards extension to middle and suchorionic zones of latticework perivillous fibrinoid; villi appear choked off by thick layers of fibrinoid that obliterate the intervillous space.

---

extending from the basal zone, into the middle and subchorial zones, in a lattice-like network. The parenchyma of MPVFD is friable, granular appearing, and dense versus the spongy and compressible texture of normal villous tissue (**Figs. 3** and **4**). Although most MPVFD results in low placental weight, due to the loss of functional and blood-filled chorionic villi, it may also be associated with a normal or even increased weight for

dates. Heavy MPVFD is generally due to the presence of abundant fibrinoid and/or proliferation of extravillous cytotrophoblast.[1,5] All forms may have regions of true chorionic villous ischemia or infarction consistent with sequelae of altered blood flow patterns and sluggish, eddy-like regions in the intervillous space, due to pathologic perivillous fibrinoid deposition. Presumably, these altered blood flow patterns also explain the

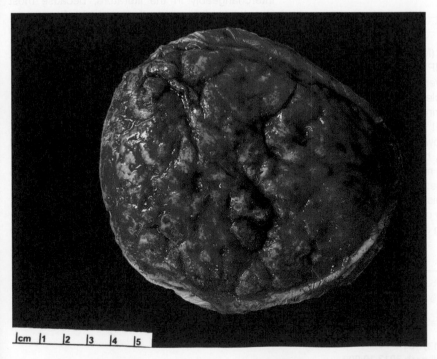

Fig. 1. Maternal surface in MPVFD. Gross image of maternal surface of placenta with MPVFD. Note the yellow-white, thickened appearance of the maternal surface.

Fig. 2. Classic MFI. Gross image of cross-sections of classic MFI with yellow-white rind of fibrinoid material seen predominantly along the basal (maternal) surface of the placenta. Note that there is also focal extension of the fibrinoid maternal into more central and subchorionic regions. (*Courtesy of Stewart Cramer, MD, University of Rochester, Rochester, NY.*)

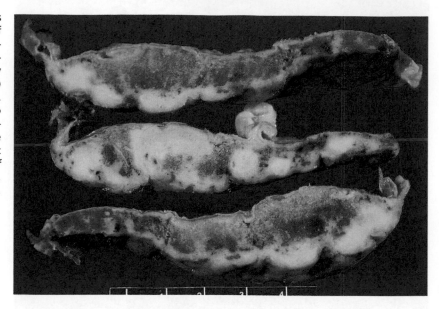

characteristic increase in extravillous trophoblast cysts (X-cell cysts) and intervillous, thrombohematomatous formation within the parenchyma (**Fig. 5**).[1] Formalin fixation highlights the pathologic fibrinoid latticework, atrophic portions of the villous tree, X-cell cysts, and thrombohematomas (see **Fig. 5**).

MICROSCOPIC FEATURES

MPVFD is characterized by marked increase in perivillous fibrinoid deposition in the intervillous space adjacent to the basal plate with varying degrees of upward extension into the midzonal and subchorionic regions (**Fig. 6**). Chorionic villi appear to stand apart, due to their circumferential sheaths of amorphous to laminated, eosinophilic fibrinoid and display varying degrees of atrophy, with loss of syncytiotrophoblast, villous vascularity, and stromal histologic detail. Although grossly, the maternal floor has a blanket-like distribution of fibrinoid, microscopically, the pathology is often discontinuous. Basal, encased, individuated villi and villous clusters, however, are matted together (so-called gitter infarct) and seem to provide scaffolding for further fibrinoid deposition (**Fig. 7**). A more extensive upward distribution is more common in placentas from later, third-trimester deliveries and is compatible with a progressive process. Excessive extravillous cytotrophoblast (X-cell) proliferations (nodular or confluent aggregations) and X-cell cysts are common, or even the

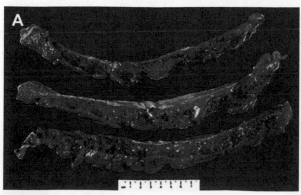

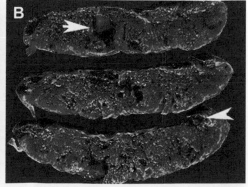

Fig. 3. Cut surfaces of placenta, normal (*A*) versus MPVFD (*B*). Gross images of cross-sections of placenta showing pale, granular and dense appearing parenchyma in MPVFD (*B*) compared with age-matched control (*A*) with more spongy and red parenchyma. Also, note intervillous thrombus (*arrow*) and chorionic cyst (*arrowhead*) within parenchyma of placenta with MPVFD.

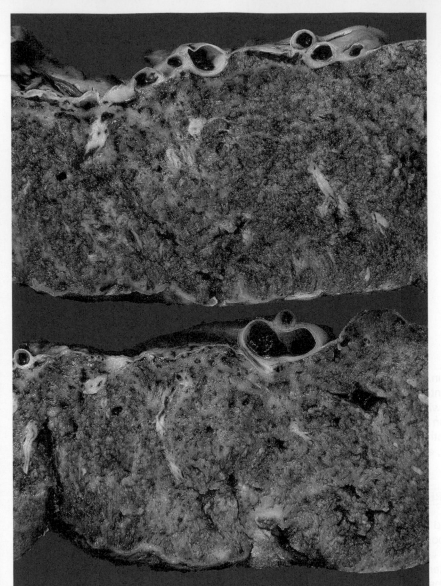

Fig. 4. Cut surfaces of placenta with MPVFD, after fixation. Closer views of gross of cross-sections of placenta showing pale, granular, and dense-appearing parenchyma in MPVFD.

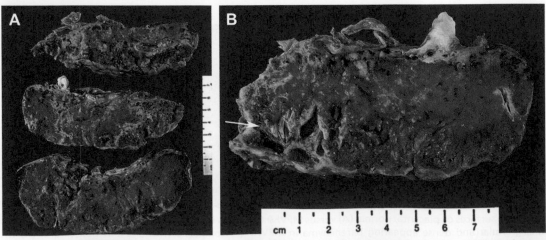

Fig. 5. Cut surfaces of placenta with MPVFD, after fixation. (*A*) Note the vertically oriented trabeculae of fibrinoid extending through the parenchyma. (*B*) Closer inspection reveals the coarse granularity of the parenchyma and an intervillous thrombus is seen (*arrow*).

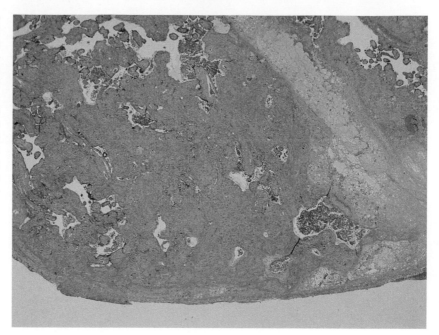

Fig. 6. Low-power photomicrograph of the basal surface (lower surface) and overlying placental parenchyma. Note the extensive perivillous fibrin deposition characterized by amorphous eosinophilic deposits that surround and choke the chorionic villi. In this image, the perivillous fibrin extends in vertical bands toward the chorionic plate (hematoxylin-eosin, original magnification ×20).

dominant, feature (**Fig. 8**). X-cell proliferations, cysts, and occasional foci of chronic chorionic villous ischemia and infarction are likely linked to development of abnormal blood flow patterns in the maternal space and sites of relative secondary ischemia. Not surprisingly, intervillous thrombohematomas may coexist or merge with areas of perivillous fibrinoid deposition. Inflammation, when present, is a minor component. Scattered lymphocytes and monocytes/histiocytes (**Fig. 9**), but not plasma cells, may be present within or adjacent to the villi. Degenerating villi may also elicit perivillous neutrophilic reactions. Lymphoplasmacytic deciduitis may occasionally be seen.[1,5,9–11]

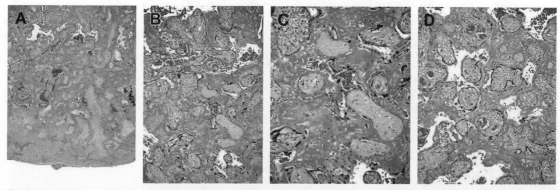

Fig. 7. Progression of MPVFD. This series of images illustrates how MPVFD is initiated near the basal surface of the placenta (*A*) and progresses toward the midzonal (*B, C*) and subchorionic regions (*D*). Notice how the villi in the basal zones ([*A*] and [*B, C* (*lower*)]) are more sclerotic than those in the midzonal region (*B, C* [*upper*]) and subchorionic region (*D*). The villi in the subchorionic region are only partially surrounded by fibrinoid and still maintain some fetal capillaries (hematoxylin-eosin, original magnifications [*A*] ×20, [*B*] ×100, [*C*] ×200, and [*D*] ×100).

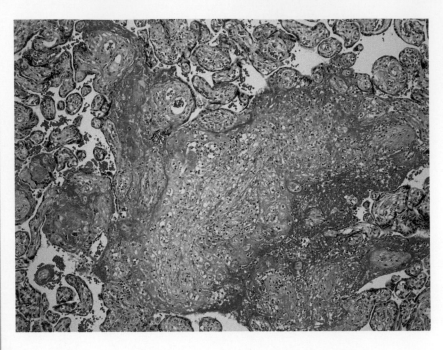

Fig. *8.* Perivillous fibrin deposition with prominent proliferation of extravillous trophoblast cells (X-cells) (hematoxylin-eosin, original magnification ×400).

DIAGNOSIS

The diagnosis of MPVFD should be suspected when the placenta is small for the gestational period, is diffusely firm, and shows a maternal

surface that is pale yellow-white and granular, and serial sections display basal deposition of granular fibrinoid material that extends upward, toward the chorionic plate in a matted and/or trabecular network. Light microscopically, basal

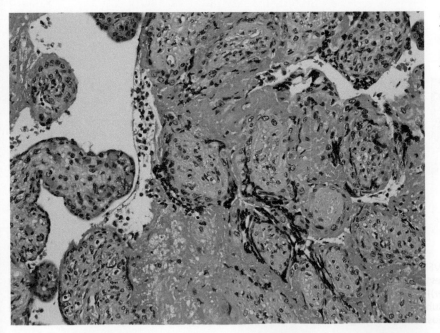

Fig. *9.* Chronic inflammatory infiltrates in MPVFD. Microscopic image of lymphohistiocytic cells within the intervillous space adjacent to areas of MPVFD. No significant chronic villitis or plasma cells are seen (hematoxylin-eosin, original magnification ×20).

chorionic villi show encasement by thick layers of perivillous fibrinoid, without the typical changes of villous ischemia. The presence of villi choked by perivillous fibrinoid is compatible with sequelae of syncytiotrophoblastic damage, and/or alterations of or imbalances among factors that maintain the normal, fluid state of the blood in the intervillous space. Syncytiotrophoblast damage is the first detectable villous change, but it is unclear if it is the initiating or merely an early event in the cascade of MPVFD.

Perivillous fibrinoid deposition is greatest in the basal zone, with variable penetration of the midchorionic and subchorionic zones. Accordingly, the authors support use of semiquantitative criteria for diagnosis of MPVFD,[7] to promote diagnostic uniformity among pathologists and particularly to help distinguish it from other lesions with fibrinoid, such as massive chronic (histiocytic noninfectious) intervillositis (MCI), until the underlying causes of these lesions are better elucidated. The authors propose that the placental pathology report should specify one of the following patterns:

1. Classic—basal villous encasement by fibrinoid along entire maternal floor and of 3 mm or greater thickness on at least one slide
2. Borderline MPVFD—involvement of 25%–50% of villi on at least one slide in transmural or nearly transmural distribution
3. Transmural MPVFD—transmural perivillous fibrinoid extension, with encasement of 50% or greater of villi on at least one slide

MPVFD may include foci of villitis and intervillositis, lymphoplasmacytic deciduitis in the extraplacental membranes or decidua basalis, and areas of ischemic change to frank infarction. The diagnosis of MPVFD, however, should be made on its predominance as the histopathologic feature (see Key Points and Differential Diagnosis). Estimates of the percentages of co-occurrence of villitis, intervillositis, and/or ischemic damage may be included in the report, especially if they are more than occasional findings, because their presence may influence treatment and frequency of clinical evaluations in subsequent pregnancies. Finally, a comment should be included indicating that MPVFD is associated with high risks for adverse perinatal outcomes and recurrence (discussed later).

DIFFERENTIAL DIAGNOSIS

The differential diagnosis includes

1. Normal perivillous fibrinoid deposition
2. Chorionic villous ischemia and infarction
3. Fetal thrombotic vasculopathy (FTV)[12–16] and other pathologies likely representing maternal alloimmune graft-versus-host disorders[17–24]
4. Diffuse chronic villitis of unknown etiology (VUE) and chronic villitis with obliterative vasculopathy/vasculitis (CVOV)[16,21]
5. MCI[25–28]

Some perivillous fibrinoid deposition is a normal feature of mature placentas[5] and likely reflects wear and tear damage to the syncytiotrophoblast. Injured trophoblast presumably releases tissue factors and/or other mediators that activate intervillous coagulation,[1] and fibrinoid plugs seal the syncytiotrophoblast defects.[5] Perivillous fibrinoid deposition, but not obliteration of the intervillous space, increases with advancing gestation. In term placentas, term stem villous surfaces show linear, thin fibrinoid profiles and patchy aggregates of perivillous deposition of laminated type of fibrin/fibrinoid (Fig. 10) that progress throughout gestation in the subchorionic, basal, and marginal zones (ie, normal regions of relatively sluggish flow and/or hypoxia, within the maternal space).[5] The main differential diagnosis for MPVFD is chorionic villous ischemic injury (including villous infarction secondary to placental bed underperfusion)[29] because perivillous fibrinoid frequently surrounds areas with loss villous viability (Fig. 11). In chorionic villous ischemia/infarction, however, increased perivillous fibrinoid deposition is concentrated around stem villi and in zones of primary, relative ischemia (discussed previously). With infarction, there is collapse of the intervillous space and syncytial knot formation and stromal loss of nuclear detail precedes syncytiotrophoblast necrosis (Fig. 12). In MPVFD, intervillous spacing is preserved and syncytiotrophoblast injury is the initial feature of villous damage.[1] Decidual arteriopathy of maternal hypertensive disorders (ie, thick-walled arterioles, atherosis, and fibrinoid necrosis) is typically absent in MPVFD.[1,9]

FTV (clusters or large areas of avascular, involuted-appearing distal terminal villi) is due to intermittent or sudden obstruction of blood flow within the villous tree. In most cases, FTV does not show perivillous fibrinoid deposition around sclerosed villi, but long-standing lesions of FTV may have foci of avascular villi with fibrinoid encasement (Fig. 13). MPVFD does not, however, display propagating thrombi or fields of chorionic villous stromal-vascular karyorrhexis with preservation of syncytiotrophoblast.[5,12,15]

Diffuse VUE and CVOV represent high-grade, destructive lymphohistiocytic villitides affecting greater than 5% of the terminal villi of midtrimester to late third-trimester placentas (32 weeks or

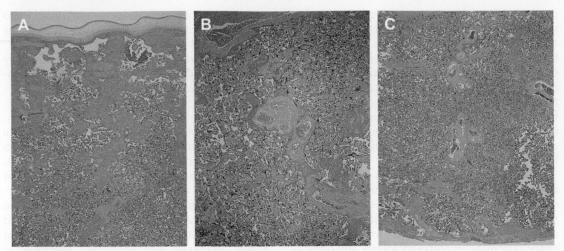

Fig. 10. Pattern of normal perivillous fibrin deposition. (*A*) Subchorionic zone with fair amount of perivillous fibrinoid deposition beneath the chorionic plate and surrounding the most proximal stem villi. (*B*) Midzonal region with small nodules of perivillous fibrinoid, which appear most prominent around stem villi. (*C*) Basal zone appears similar to midzonal region with small nodules of perivillous fibrinoid, especially around stem villi. Only a small amount of perivillous fibrinoid is noted directly adjacent to the basal plate (hematoxylin-eosin, original magnifications [*A*] ×20, [*B*] ×40, and [*C*] ×20).

greater of gestation) with perivillous fibrinoid deposition around individual and clusters of chorionic villi (see **Fig. 13**). CVOV also affects distal stem villi and includes villous lymphohistiocytic vasculitis and thrombosis. Both show variable presence of lymphoplasmacytic deciduitis and chronic chorioamnionitis and may include a prominent component of perivillous fibrinoid deposition.[15,16,21,30] MPVFD displays scant foci of chronic villitis and

no chorionic villous stem vessel vasculitis or thrombosis.

MCI is characterized by diffuse mononuclear infiltrates (lymphocytes, monocytes, and histiocytes) in the intervillous space, the essential absence of villitis, and may show mild villous and intervillous fibrinoid deposition.[8] Literature on this lesion is inconsistent, however. In a recent study, Parant and colleagues[28] defined the severe

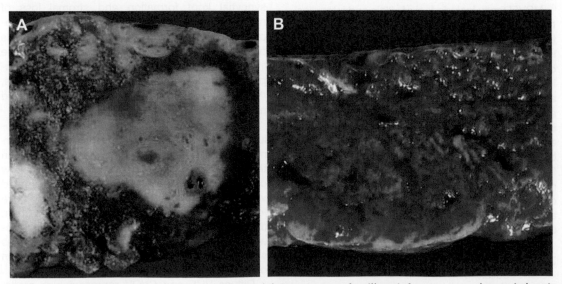

Fig. 11. Gross comparison of infarction and MPVFD. (*A*) Gross image of a villous infarction secondary to ischemia. Note the wedge-shaped lesion with a tan homogeneous, firm cut surface and well-defined borders. Compare with gross image of MPVFD (*B*), which shows more diffuse involvement of the parenchyma with linear and small nodular accumulations of fibrinoid but no formation of a well-defined lesion.

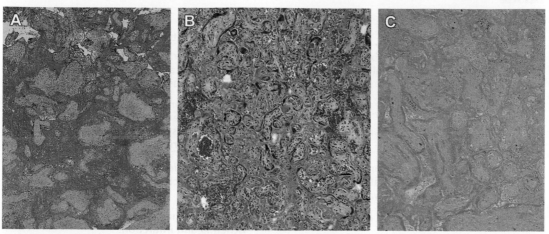

Fig. 12. Differential diagnosis of MPVFD-comparison of MPVFD and infarction. (*A*) MPVFD, (*B*) subacute infarction, and (*C*) remote infarction. Note that in MPVFD the intervillous space is filled with fibrinoid, but the spacing between the villi is preserved, and in infarction there is collapse of the intervillous space. Note also the presence of coagulative necrosis of villi in infarct compared with the more fibrotic but not necrotic villi of MPVFD (hematoxylin-eosin, original magnifications [*A*] ×100, [*B*] ×200, and [*C*] ×200).

category of pathology of chronic intervillositis of unknown etiology (with greater than 50% of the intervillous space on the slide showing infiltrate) as also including "massive and confluent perivillous fibrinoid with *mild* mononuclear infiltrate."

Thus, the authors propose that the diagnosis of MPVFD and other lesions be based on the predominant, histopathologic feature and that any secondary feature be included as a modifier and semiquantitated.

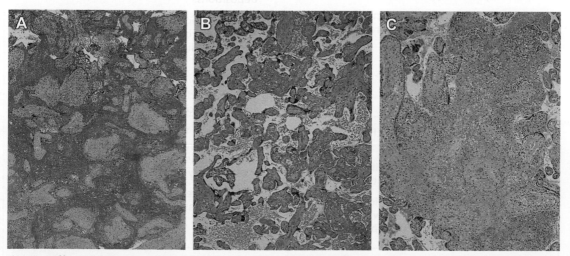

Fig. 13. Differential diagnosis of MPVFD—comparison of MPVFD with FTV/avascular villi and chronic villitis/VUE. (*A*) MPVFD, (*B*) FTV/avascular villi, and (*C*) chronic villitis/VUE. In FTV, avascular villi (*B*) are characterized by sclerotic-appearing villi with preservation of the intervillous space; however, the villi can become encircled in small amounts of perivillous fibrinoid. Stem villous or chorionic thrombi, which can accompany avascular villi, are typically not seen in MPVFD. In chronic villitis/VUE (*C*), there is perivillous fibrinoid deposition associated with villous agglutination and chronic inflammation. MPVFD does not typically show agglutination of villi or significant chronic inflammation of villous parenchyma (hematoxylin-eosin, original magnifications [*A–C*] ×100).

Differential Diagnosis
OF MPVFD

ΔΔ

MPVFD	Differential Entity
1. Distal chorionic villous tree branches are diffusely choked and normally to widely spaced by thick layers of fibrinoid	Normal-term perivillous fibrinoid 1. Deposition is around scattered stem villi, in thin profiles. 2. Perivillous fibrinoid is a thin layer in relatively ischemic zone of basal and subchorionic villi; terminal villi show occasional aggregates as intervillous bridges.
1. Grossly, a permeative network of fibrinous material is seen based at maternal surface and branching upwards toward chorionic plate. 2. Chorionic villous ischemia is a minor finding 3. Distal chorionic villous tree branches are diffusely choked, and normally to widely spaced, by thick layers of fibrinoid 4. Atherosis/fibrinoid necrosis is not seen unless there is a complicating comorbidity of underlying maternal hypertension or thrombophilia 5. MPVFD shows no necrosis of decidua of extraplacental membranes unless there is a comorbid condition of hypertension or primary disorder with vasculopathy	Chronic chorionic villous ischemia/infarction 1. Grossly, infarctions are triangular shaped or rounded. 2. The Predominant feature is chorionic villous ischemia and infarction. 3. Villi show crowding with thin layers of intervening fibrinoid deposition. 4. Decidual arteriopathy is a feature in ischemia-induced pathology due to placental bed under perfusion. 5. Decidual laminar-like or leukocytoclastic necrosis in membranes is often present.
1. Sampling artifact is much less of an issue, because basal distribution of fibrinoid is blanket-like grossly and 2. Distal chorionic villous tree branches are diffusely choked and normally to widely spaced by thick layers of fibrinoid 3. MPVFD does not show chorionic plate or stem villous and/or propagating thrombosis.	FTV 1. Sampling affects detection of chorionic plate or stem villous thrombi and distal villous sclerosis in cases of FTV, and sampling artifact may lead to errors in interpretation of small perivillous fibrinoid depositions. 2. Characteristically, FTV shows scant to no perivillous fibrinoid deposition around sclerosed villi; the sclerosed villi remain isolated and free floating. 3. Occasionally, presumably long-standing clusters of sclerotic villi of FTV may show fibrinoid encasement.
1. MFPVD shows foci or patchy chronic villitis and intervillositis. 2. MPVFD does not show stem villous vasculitis/thrombosis as a dominant feature. 3. The occasional focus of chronic villitis or intervillositis may reflect an overlap in aspects of pathologic mechanisms or pathways leading to DVUE, CVOV, and MPVFD.	Diffuse chronic VUE and CVOV 1. The dominant histopathologic pattern is diffuse villitis and/or obliterative vasculitis/vasculopathy. 2. CVOV has stem villous vasculitis or thrombosis as a dominant feature.
1. MPVD can contain foci or patchy presence of chronic lymphocytic/monocytic intervillositis. 2. The occasional focus of chronic intervillositis may reflect an overlap in aspects of pathologic mechanisms or triggers of pathways leading to MCI and MPVFD, respectively.	MCI 1. MCI is diffusely present in all zones of the maternal space (subchorionic, middle, and basal).

IMPACT AND UPDATES IN PATHOGENESIS

MPVFD is associated with high rates of adverse perinatal outcomes, such as prematurity (preterm delivery in 26%–60%), intrauterine growth restriction (24%–100%), spontaneous abortion, stillbirth (13%–50%), neonatal death, and long-term neurologic impairment.[3,4,31–34] Women delivering placentas with MPVFD more frequently have poor past reproductive histories (with or without documented placental examination).[4,35] Studies have correspondingly revealed that MPVFD exhibits high recurrence risks (12%–78%),[2–4,7,35–37] with earlier onset and more rapid progression by ultrasonographic examination.[2,4,11,31] Prenatal, ultrasonographic findings of oligohydramnios; fetal intrauterine growth restriction (especially early onset); and a dense, hypoechogenic placenta have been noted as strongly suggestive of MPVFD,[31] but Uxa and colleagues[38] did not find these a consistent constellation of antenatal features. The classic triad, however, of these ultrasonographic findings may reflect the onset, extent, and rapidity of fibrinoid deposition, period of gestation, and compromise of fetal renal blood flow due to hypovolemia associated with decline in placental function. Taweevisit and Thorner[39] linked MPVFD, fetal cystic renal dysplasia, and oligohydramnios and suggested that fetoplacental factors may also play a role in the pathogenesis of MPVFD, possibly through alterations in uterine hydrostatic pressure gradients.

As discussed previously, the causes of the excessive accumulations of amorphous fibrinoid material encasing chorionic villi and features of loss of syncytiotrophoblast viability are incompletely understood. Elements of the maternal blood and trophoblast-generated procoagulant and anticoagulant molecules and matrix contribute to a normal villous surface and maintenance of a fluid intervillous space. The amorphous, perivillous material, normally present in the intervillous space, immunohistochemically and ultrastructurally appears to be a combination of serum fibrin of the maternal coagulation cascade (a laminated fibrin-type fibrinoid) and trophoblast-derived extracellular substance (matrix-predominant type fibrinoid).[5–7,9,10,40] Abnormal amounts of fibrin or fibrinoid dominant deposition may partly reflect the relative numbers of proliferating or neighboring cytotrophoblasts and decidual cells.[1]

The microscopic features of MPVFD are highly suggestive of either direct damage to the syncytiotrophoblast and/or disturbances in the balance of dually derived intervillous procoagulant/anticoagulant factors necessary to maintain the fluid state of the blood in the maternal space. To date, there is evidence that at least some MPVFD represents sequelae of a maternal autoimmune or alloimmune condition. In addition to its high risks of recurrence,

1. MPVFD is more common in women antiphospholipid (APL) antibody syndrome and other autoimmune disorders with or without thrombophilia.[8,41–45]
2. Women with a prior diagnosis of MPVFD and APL syndrome, treated with intravenous immunoglobulin, have had improved pregnancy outcomes.[44]
3. MPVFD may be discordant in dichorionic[9] or monochorionic[2] twin placentas.
4. MPVFD may coexist with chronic intervillositis.[28,46]

The syncytiotrophoblast may be the primary target of maternal antitrophoblast antibodies[47] and release factors, such as tissue necrosis factor or Hageman factor, that activate coagulation. Somewhat challenging is the observation that MPVFD may be associated with maternal primary hypertension and preeclampsia.[4,37,48] These associations, however, may represent overlap among maternal risk factors for MPVFD and hypertension, because hypertensive disorders and APL syndrome can co-occur. Alternatively, the sequelae of trophoblastic or villous hypoxic damage could result in confounding activation of abnormal coagulation in the intervillous space[1,5] and potentiate an otherwise insignificant or low-grade trophoblastic abnormality or process of fibrinoid deposition.

As a corollary to the above discussion, MPFVD has also been linked to primary maternal inherited coagulation factor deficiencies and abnormalities[45,49–51] and long-chain 3-hydroxyacyl-CoA dehydrogenase (LCHAD) deficiency[52] with mutations in LCHAD gene.[53] Thus, blood flow in the maternal space may become compromised by an intervillous process initiated by imbalances among the components and activities of the intervillous procoagulant/anticoagulant factors. Women, with or without an underlying autoimmune disease but with a history of a prior pregnancy complicated by a placental diagnosis of MPVFD, who were treated with low-dose heparin and aspirin during their subsequent pregnancies have had improved gestational outcomes.[54] Anticoagulant therapy may prove to be protective against the recurrence or severity of MPVFD.

In conclusion, the fibrinoid deposition of MPVFD likely represents the outcome of a final common pathway potentially triggered by a variety of conditions or pathologies that disturb the normal and inducible factors that maintain the integrity of the

Pitfalls

Massive perivillous fibrinoid deposition/MFI	! Most common misdiagnosis is chorionic villous ischemia/infarction.

Massive perivillous fibrinoid deposition/MFI

! Most common misdiagnosis is chorionic villous ischemia/infarction.

- Grossly placental bed ischemia due to maternal vascular disease creates triangular-shaped or rounded masses of infarcted villi whose broadest aspects lie along maternal surface; MPVFD has a diffuse pattern of distribution of fibrinoid along basal plate.

- Chorionic villous ischemia shows thin layers of intervening fibrinoid deposition or small, nodular excrescences that bridge to other villi and predominantly involves stem villi and subchorionic regions. MPVFD isolates chorionic villi and obliterates intervillous space, from basal plate upward.

- Infarction displays collapse of the intervillous space with fibrinoid deposition and villous necrosis. MPVFD shows individuated villi surrounded by fibrin without coagulative necrosis.

- MPVFD can result in abnormal channels of blood flow in maternal space and create zones of ischemia that compromise chorionic villi and result in foci of infarction.

! MPVD can contain foci of chronic villitis and MCI.

- The occasional focus of chronic intervillositis may reflect an overlap in the portions of pathologic pathways between MCI and MPVFD.

! MPFVD may show rare focus of chorionic villous thrombosis.

syncytiotrophoblast and the fluidity of blood in the maternal space. Ongoing damage and accelerating compromise of the blood flow within the intervillous space may obscure the inciting pathology or combine with elements of chronic villitis. The triggers, however, are likely potent and/or in high concentrations, because they seem to irreversibly commit the perivillous space to a process of marked fibrinoid deposition and accumulation. The rarity of MPVFD suggests that there are many sites of duplication within the normal villous protective and reparative systems, which guard against pathologic amounts of fibrinoid deposition.[55–57]

REFERENCES

1. Faye-Petersen O, Heller D, Joshi V. Handbook of placental pathology. 2nd edtion. Oxford (United Kingdom): Taylor & Francis; 2006. 53–110.
2. Bane AL, Gillan JE. Massive perivillous fibrinoid causing recurrent placental failure. BJOG 2003; 110:292–5.
3. Andres RL, Kuyper W, Resnik R, et al. The association of maternal floor infarction of the placenta with adverse perinatal outcome. Am J Obstet Gynecol 1990;163:935–8.
4. Naeye RL. Maternal floor infarction. Hum Pathol 1985;16:823–8.
5. Baergen R. Manual of pathology of the human placenta. 2nd edition. New York: Springer; 2011. p. 335–427.
6. Fox H, Elston CW. Pathology of the placenta. Major Probl Pathol 1978;7:1–491.
7. Katzman PJ, Genest DR. Maternal floor infarction and massive perivillous fibrin deposition: histological definitions, association with intrauterine fetal growth restriction, and risk of recurrence. Pediatr Dev Pathol 2002;5:159–64.
8. Sebire NJ, Backos M, Goldin RD, et al. Placental massive perivillous fibrin deposition associated with antiphospholipid antibody syndrome. BJOG 2002;109:570–3.
9. Redline RW, Jiang JG, Shah D. Discordancy for maternal floor infarction in dizygotic twin placentas. Hum Pathol 2003;34:822–4.
10. Vernof KK, Benirschke K, Kephart GM, et al. Maternal floor infarction: relationship to X cells, major basic protein, and adverse perinatal outcome. Am J Obstet Gynecol 1992;167:1355–63.
11. Mandsager NT, Bendon R, Mostello D, et al. Maternal floor infarction of the placenta: prenatal diagnosis and clinical significance. Obstet Gynecol 1994;83:750–4.

12. Redline RW, Pappin A. Fetal thrombotic vasculopathy: the clinical significance of extensive avascular villi. Hum Pathol 1995;26:80–5.

13. Kraus FT. Placenta: thrombosis of fetal stem vessels with fetal thrombotic vasculopathy and chronic villitis. Pediatr Pathol Lab Med 1996;16:143–8.

14. Kraus FT, Acheen VI. Fetal thrombotic vasculopathy in the placenta: cerebral thrombi and infarcts, coagulopathies, and cerebral palsy. Hum Pathol 1999; 30:759–69.

15. Faye-Petersen O, Reilly S. Demystifying the pathologic diagnoses of villitis and fetal thrombotic vasculopathy. Available at: http://neoreviews.aap publications.org/cgi/content/full/neoreviews;9/9/e399. 2008.

16. Redline RW. Disorders of placental circulation and the fetal brain. Clin Perinatol 2009;36:549–59.

17. Knox WF, Fox H. Villitis of unknown aetiology: its incidence and significance in placentae from a British population. Placenta 1984;5:395–402.

18. Redline RW, Abramowsky CR. Clinical and pathologic aspects of recurrent placental villitis. Hum Pathol 1985;16:727–31.

19. Redline RW, Patterson P. Villitis of unknown etiology is associated with major infiltration of fetal tissue by maternal inflammatory cells. Am J Pathol 1993;143: 473–9.

20. Myerson D, Parkin RK, Benirschke K, et al. The pathogenesis of villitis of unknown etiology: analysis with a new conjoint immunohistochemistry-in situ hybridization procedure to identify specific maternal and fetal cells. Pediatr Dev Pathol 2006;9:257–65.

21. Redline RW. Villitis of unknown etiology: noninfectious chronic villitis in the placenta. Hum Pathol 2007;38:1439–46.

22. Boog G. Chronic villitis of unknown etiology. Eur J Obstet Gynecol Reprod Biol 2008;136:9–15.

23. Kim JS, Romero R, Kim MR, et al. Involvement of Hofbauer cells and maternal T cells in villitis of unknown aetiology. Histopathology 2008;52:457–64.

24. Tang Z, Abrahams VM, Mor G, et al. Placental Hofbauer cells and complications of pregnancy. Ann N Y Acad Sci 2011;1221:103–8.

25. Labarrere C, Mullen E. Fibrinoid and trophoblastic necrosis with massive chronic intervillositis: an extreme variant of villitis of unknown etiology. Am J Reprod Immunol Microbiol 1987;15:85–91.

26. Doss BJ, Greene MF, Hill J, et al. Massive chronic intervillositis associated with recurrent abortions. Hum Pathol 1995;26:1245–51.

27. Boyd TK, Redline RW. Chronic histiocytic intervillositis: a placental lesion associated with recurrent reproductive loss. Hum Pathol 2000;31:1389–96.

28. Parant O, Capdet J, Kessler S, et al. Chronic intervillositis of unknown etiology (CIUE): relation between placental lesions and perinatal outcome. Eur J Obstet Gynecol Reprod Biol 2009;143:9–13.

29. Sun CC, Revell VO, Belli AJ, et al. Discrepancy in pathologic diagnosis of placental lesions. Arch Pathol Lab Med 2002;126:706–9.

30. Redline RW. Severe fetal placental vascular lesions in term infants with neurologic impairment. Am J Obstet Gynecol 2005;192:452–7.

31. Clewell WH, Manchester DK. Recurrent maternal floor infarction: a preventable cause of fetal death. Am J Obstet Gynecol 1983;147:346–7.

32. Nickel RE. Maternal floor infarction: an unusual cause of intrauterine growth retardation. Am J Dis Child 1988;142:1270–1.

33. Adams-Chapman I, Vaucher YE, Bejar RF, et al. Maternal floor infarction of the placenta: association with central nervous system injury and adverse neurodevelopmental outcome. J Perinatol 2002;22: 236–41.

34. Waters BL, Ashikaga T. Significance of perivillous fibrin/oid deposition in uterine evacuation specimens. Am J Surg Pathol 2006;30:760–5.

35. Benirschke K, Kaufmann P, Baergen R. Pathology of the human placenta. 5th edition. New York: Springer; 2006.

36. Redline RW. Maternal floor infarction and massive perivillous fibrin deposition: clinicopathologic entities in flux. Adv Anat Pathol 2002;9:372–3.

37. Fuke Y, Aono T, Imai S, et al. Clinical significance and treatment of massive intervillous fibrin deposition associated with recurrent fetal growth retardation. Gynecol Obstet Invest 1994;38:5–9.

38. Uxa R, Baczyk D, Kingdom JC, et al. Genetic polymorphisms in the fibrinolytic system of placentas with massive perivillous fibrin deposition. Placenta 2010;31:499–505.

39. Taweevisit M, Thorner PS. Maternal floor infarction associated with oligohydramnios and cystic renal dysplasia: report of 2 cases. Pediatr Dev Pathol 2010;13:116–20.

40. Frank HG, Malekzadeh F, Kertschanska S, et al. Immunohistochemistry of two different types of placental fibrinoid. Acta Anat 1994;150:55–68.

41. Hung NA, Jackson C, Nicholson M, et al. Pregnancy-related polymyositis and massive perivillous fibrin deposition in the placenta: are they pathogenetically related? Arthritis Rheum 2006;55: 154–6.

42. Bendon RW, Hommel AB. Maternal floor infarction in autoimmune disease: two cases. Pediatr Pathol Lab Med 1996;16:293–7.

43. Sebire NJ, Backos M, El Gaddal S, et al. Placental pathology, antiphospholipid antibodies, and pregnancy outcome in recurrent miscarriage patients. Obstet Gynecol 2003;101:258–63.

44. Chang P, Millar D, Tsang P, et al. Intravenous immunoglobulin in antiphospholipid syndrome and maternal floor infarction when standard treatment fails: a case report. Am J Perinatol 2006;23:125–9.

45. Gogia N, Machin GA. Maternal thrombophilias are associated with specific placental lesions. Pediatr Dev Pathol 2008;11:424–9.

46. Weber MA, Nikkels PG, Hamoen K, et al. Co-occurrence of massive perivillous fibrin deposition and chronic intervillositis: case report. Pediatr Dev Pathol 2006;9:234–8.

47. McCrae KR, DeMichele AM, Pandhi P, et al. Detection of antitrophoblast antibodies in the sera of patients with anticardiolipin antibodies and fetal loss. Blood 1993;82:2730–41.

48. Lindoff C, Astedt B. Plasminogen activator of urokinase type and its inhibitor of placental type in hypertensive pregnancies and in intrauterine growth retardation: possible markers of placental function. Am J Obstet Gynecol 1994;171:60–4.

49. Raspollini MR, Oliva E, Roberts DJ. Placental histopathologic features in patients with thrombophilic mutations. J Matern Fetal Neonatal Med 2007;20: 113–23.

50. Katz VL, DiTomasso J, Farmer R, et al. Activated protein C resistance associated with maternal floor infarction treated with low-molecular-weight heparin. Am J Perinatol 2002;19:273–7.

51. Svensson AM, Waters BL, Laszik ZG, et al. The protein C system in placental massive perivillous fibrin deposition. Blood Coagul Fibrinolysis 2004; 15:491–5.

52. Matern D, Schehata BM, Shekhawa P, et al. Placental floor infarction complicating the pregnancy of a fetus with long-chain 3-hydroxyacyl-CoA dehydrogenase (LCHAD) deficiency. Mol Genet Metab 2001;72:265–8.

53. Carruth A, Strauss A, Bennett M, et al. Mutations in long-chain 3-Hydroxyacyl-CoA dehydrogenase and placental maternal floor infarct/massive perivillous fibrin deposition. Pediatr Dev Pathol 2010; 13:138.

54. Makino A, Suzuki Y, Yamamoto T, et al. Use of aspirin and low-molecular-weight heparin to prevent recurrence of maternal floor infarction in women without evidence of antiphospholipid antibody syndrome. Fetal Diagn Ther 2004;19:261–5.

55. Katz VL, Bowes WA Jr, Sierkh AE. Maternal floor infarction of the placenta associated with elevated second trimester serum alpha-fetoprotein. Am J Perinatol 1987;4:225–8.

56. Robinson L, Grau P, Crandall BF. Pregnancy outcomes after increasing maternal serum alpha-fetoprotein levels. Obstet Gynecol 1989;74: 17–20.

57. Gorbe E, Rigo J Jr, Marton T, et al. "Maternal floor infarct", simultaneous manifestation of intrauterine fetal retardation and high maternal AFP level. Z Geburtshilfe Neonatol 1999;203:218–20 [in German].

Villitis of Unknown Etiology and Massive Chronic Intervillositis

Joanna S.Y. Chan, MD

KEYWORDS

• Villitis of unknown etiology • Villitis • Intervillositis • Intervillitis • Massive chronic intervillositis
• Chronic histiocytic intervillositis

ABSTRACT

Villitis of unknown etiology (VUE) is a common lesion affecting from 6.6% to 33.8% of third-trimester placentas. VUE needs to be distinguished from villitis of infectious etiology, most commonly cytomegalovirus and syphilis. Clinically, this lesion is associated with intrauterine growth retardation, intrauterine fetal demise, fetal neural impairment, maternal alloimmune and autoimmune disease, and maternal hypertension. It has a tendency to recur in subsequent pregnancies. Massive chronic intervillositis (MCI), also known as chronic histiocytic intervillositis, is a rare lesion that has an unclear relationship with VUE. MCI is associated with recurrent abortions.

VILLITIS OF UNKNOWN ETIOLOGY

VUE is a common lesion affecting from 6.6% to 33.8% of third-trimester placentas.[1–3] Unfortunately, there is both high intraobserver and interobserver variability in making this diagnosis.[4] VUE needs to be distinguished from villitis of infectious etiology, the most common causes of which are rubella, syphilis, *Toxoplasma gondii*, and cytomegalovirus.[3] Histologically, it is characterized by a diffuse villous inflammatory infiltrate, which is usually lymphohistiocytic in nature.[5] VUE may be associated with fetal vascular thrombotic lesions, which in combination is a strong risk factor for a poor fetal outcome.[6–8] Clinically, this lesion is associated with intrauterine growth retardation (IUGR),[9–11] intrauterine fetal demise, fetal neural impairment,[6] maternal alloimmune

Key Features
OF VILLITIS OF UNKNOWN ETIOLOGY

Clinical

• History of villitis of unknown etiology (VUE)

• Maternal history of autoimmune disease or donor ovum

• No apparent infection of mother or neonate

Gross Pathology

• No definitive gross lesion

• May be pale or stiff

Histology

• Patchy villous involvement

• Villi expanded by lymphohistiocytic infiltrate

• Villous vessels may be involved by inflammatory cells

and autoimmune disease,[12,13] and maternal hypertension or preeclampsia.[14,15] More recent studies have also shown an association between VUE and donated ovum during in vitro fertilization.[16,17] There is a high recurrence rate of VUE in successive pregnancies, particularly with the same father.[18] VUE is not usually associated with any gross or macroscopic lesions. Although an affected placenta may occasionally be paler or firmer than usual due to increased fibrin, this is indistinguishable from increased perivillous

Disclosures: None.
Department of Pathology, Anatomy, and Cell Biology; Thomas Jefferson University Hospital; 132 South 10th Street, Main Building; Philadelphia, PA 19123
E-mail address: joanna.chan@jefferson.edu

Surgical Pathology 6 (2013) 115–126
http://dx.doi.org/10.1016/j.path.2012.11.004
1875-9181/13/$ – see front matter © 2013 Elsevier Inc. All rights reserved.

surgpath.theclinics.com

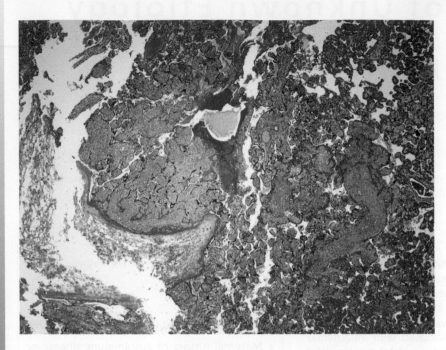

Fig. 1. VUE (H&E, 4×).

fibrin deposition of any other etiology.[5,19] In extensive cases of VUE with associated necrosis, the villous tissue may appear mottled.[19] Microscopically, the villi are invaded and expanded by a mononuclear infiltrate (**Fig. 1**). This infiltrate is usually lymphohistiocytic (**Fig. 2**); however, occasionally it is purely lymphocytic or histiocytic (**Fig. 3**). Rarely, in a purely histiocytic infiltrate, giant cells can be identified (**Fig. 4**).[5] This inflammation

can be associated with vascular obliteration and thrombosis as well as avascular villi (**Fig. 5**) and villous stromal karyorrhexis (**Fig. 6**).[5,8] VUE is most commonly found in a patchy pattern, usually involving no more than 10 villi per focus. It is often present in a parabasal pattern with associated villitis of anchoring villi (**Fig. 7**); however, it can be found more randomly distributed throughout the placenta with no relationship to the basal plate.[5]

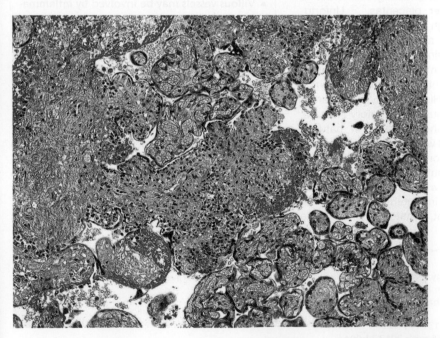

Fig. 2. Lymphohistiocytic infiltrate in VUE (H&E, 20×).

Fig. 3. Lymphocytic infiltrate in VUE (H&E, 20×).

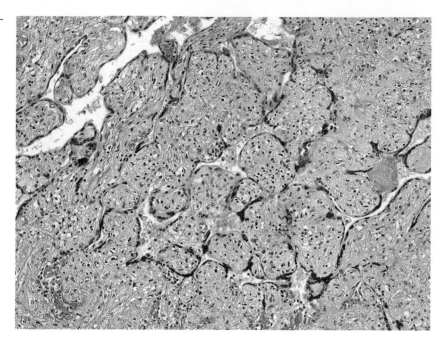

DIAGNOSIS AND DIFFERENTIAL DIAGNOSIS OF VILLITIS OF UNKNOWN ETIOLOGY

The most important differential in the diagnosis of VUE is to distinguish it from villitis of infectious origin. This is most easily done with clinical history. The most common causes of infectious chronic villitis are *Treponema pallidum*, cytomegalovirus, *Toxoplasma gondii*, and rubella,[3] although the incidence of rubella has decreased dramatically with the prevalence of childhood vaccination. Other infectious causes include *Mycobacterium tuberculosis*,[20] *Listeria monocytogenes*,[21] *Klebsiella pneumonia*,[22] *Varicella zoster*,[23] *Trypanosoma*

Fig. 4. Giant cell in VUE, (H&E, 20×).

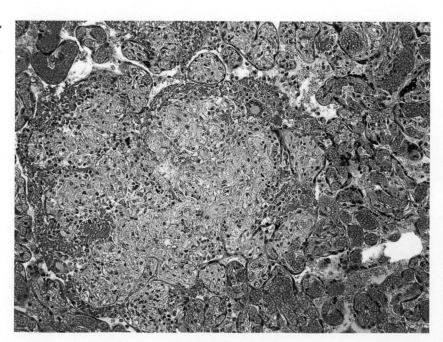

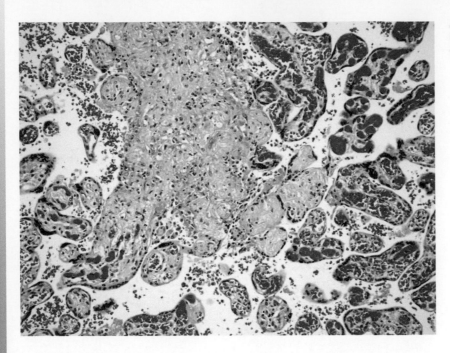

Fig. 5. Avascular villi in various stages of hyalinization, (H&E, 20×).

cruzi,[24] parvovirus, herpes simplex virus,[25] and candida species.[26] Special stains for infectious agents, such as Gram stain or Gomori methanamine silver (GMS) stain, may be useful in identifying microorganisms when there is clinical suspicion. Some infectious causes have specific histologic findings, such as the owl-eye nuclear inclusion of cytomegalovirus (**Fig. 8**) or lantern cells of parvovirus (**Fig. 9**),[19] which are pathognomonic for an infectious cause. The presence of the actual infectious organism is also pathognomonic for infectious disease, such as *Toxoplasma* cysts (**Fig. 10**). In the absence of clinical history and specific histology indicating infection, there are

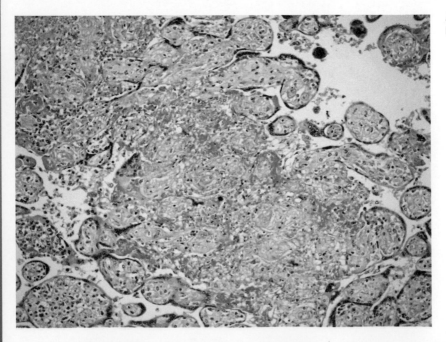

Fig. 6. Villous stromal karyorrhexis, (H&E, 20×).

Fig. 7. VUE associated with maternal surface, (H&E, 10×).

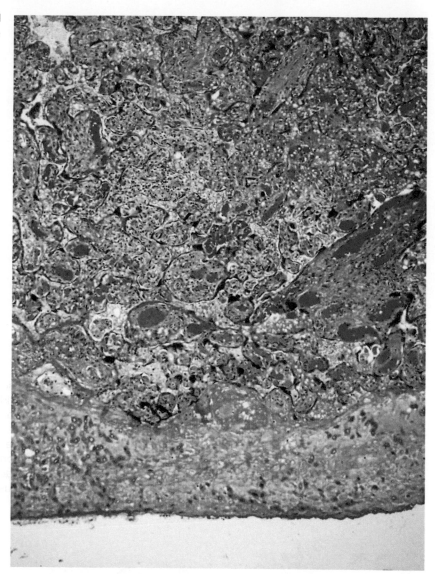

also some general histologic features that may also suggest an infectious etiology. Infectious villitis is usually a diffuse process involving all areas of the placenta, including most of the placental villous tissue as well as the umbilical cord, chorionic plate, and extraplacental membranes. Placentas with infectious villitis usually also show evidence of long standing inflammation, as evidenced by having villous fibrosis and calcification, as opposed to VUE's more acute findings of fibrinoid deposition and necrosis.[3] These findings are summarized in **Table 1**. Histologic findings must be carefully correlated with clinical history, because some causes of infectious villitis, in particular syphilis, are difficult to distinguish from VUE. Infectious causes, however, can never be

completely excluded. Villi with inflammatory cells can also be associated with ischemic placental lesions, such as infarcts, and should not be diagnosed as VUE.[19] Other entities in the differential diagnosis of VUE are decidual necrosis, acute villitis, maternal floor infarction (massive perivillous fibrin deposition), massive chronic intervillositis (MCI), and chorioamnionitis.

The focal nature of VUE dictates that the diagnosis of VUE requires thorough sampling of the placenta. It has been suggested that 4 to 6 sections of placenta need to be examined to detect up to 90% of cases of VUE.[2,27] As discussed previously, VUE is most often located in the basal plate, so care must be taken to sample the maternal surface, taking full-thickness sections that include the

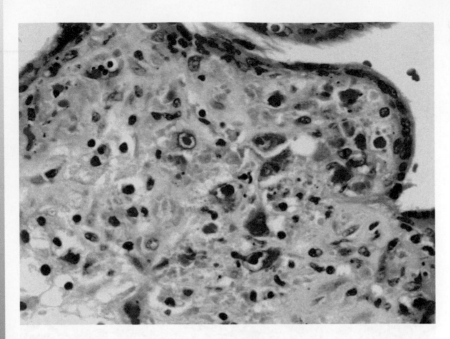

Fig. 8. CMV inclusion, (H&E, 40×).

maternal surface as well as possibly submitting sections that contain additional sections of maternal surface only. A diagnosis of VUE is often suggested at low-power magnification (<10×) using hematoxylin-eosin (H&E) staining, in which the involved villi are expanded and more cellular compared with surrounding villous tissue. When the inflammatory cells of VUE involve the villous vasculature, there is also often associated villous vascular thrombosis, evidenced by villous stromal karyorrhexis, stromal fibrosis, and avascular villi.[6] The severity of villitis can appear on a spectrum, ranging from mild to severe. Mild villitis is diagnosed when there are only a few lesions per full-thickness section of placenta with no more than one inflammatory focus per low-power field.

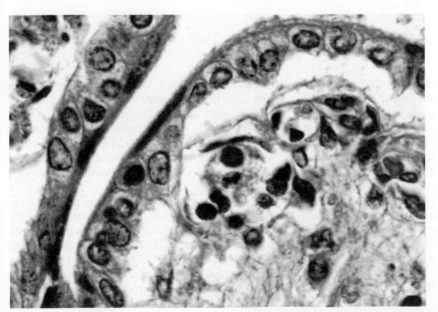

Fig. 9. Parvovirus inclusion, (H&E, 80×).

Fig. 10. Toxoplasma cyst, (H&E, 20×).

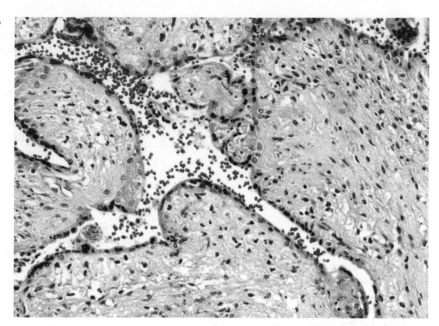

Moderate villitis can involve up to 25% of the placental villous tissue examined, whereas severe villitis is diffuse, involving greater than 25% of the placenta.[5] The severity of VUE should be reported when making the diagnosis. In both VUE and MCI, there is no role for immunohistochemical examination of the inflammatory cells. Both infectious villitis and VUE tend to consist of mostly macrophages and CD8+ T cells.[28] Because VUE is so prevalent, immunohistochemical or special stains should not

Table 1 Infectious villitis versus VUE		
	Infectious Villitis	**VUE**
Incidence	Extremely rare	Relatively common
Clinical maternal	History of Infection	Obesity Lower socioeconomic status Gestational hypertension Preeclampsia Donor ovum
Stage of pregnancy	Premature	>32-Wk gestation
Recurrence	Rare	10%–15%
Severity in recurrence	Less than original	Greater than original
Fetal infection	Yes	No
Placental involvement	Umbilical cord Chorionic plate Extraplacental membranes	Terminal and stem villi only
Villous involvement	Diffuse	Focal
Duration of villitis	Long-standing with fibrosis and calcification	Recent with fibrin and necrosis
Specific histologic findings	Infection specific (eg, owl-eye inclusion of CMV)	No specific findings
Microorganisms	May be identified by H&E or special stains (Gram stain, GMS)	None identified

Pitfalls
IN DIAGNOSIS OF **VUE**

Infectious villitis

! Clinical history of maternal or neonatal infection

! Presence of acute inflammation/abscesses

! Specific infectious findings

Infarction

! Inflammatory cells in close proximity to infarcted villi

be used in standard diagnosis. If the lesion is histologically consistent with infectious villitis (discussed previously) or there is a clinical history of infection, then a Gram stain or immunohistochemical stain for the most common infectious organisms may be indicated.

ETIOLOGY OF VUE

There are two main hypotheses for the origin of VUE, namely an unidentified infection and an immunologically mediated graft-versus-host reaction. Most recent studies seem to support the graft-versus-host hypothesis. Evidence against an unidentified infectious cause includes probing placentas with VUE using polymerase chain reaction for universal bacterial 16S ribosomal RNA DNA that was negative, decreasing the likelihood of bacterial infection, subclinical or otherwise.[29] Another factor that decreases the possibility of an infectious cause is the observation that, despite extensive study with increasingly sophisticated diagnostic techniques, the incidence of VUE has not significantly decreased with increased detection of infectious particles. Study of the chemokines associated with VUE compared with the chemokines in placentas with an infectious inflammatory response showed that VUE has a different chemokine profile, again suggesting that VUE is not of infectious origin.[30] Unrecognized viral infections are difficult to completely rule out, however, because viruses can be subtle to diagnose and be present without clinical presentation in the neonate or mother.[5,28] Characterization of the inflammatory infiltrate shows that the lymphocytes are of maternal origin and the histiocytes are fetally derived.[30–34] Although this does not rule out the possibility of a maternal response to an infectious agent presented by fetal macrophages, it decreases the possibility of VUE

being a reaction to a fetal infection. The graft-versus-host reaction hypothesis was first created in response to the observation that there were high levels of recurrence of VUE in successive pregnancies with the same father as well as the observation that the severity of VUE also increased with successive pregnancies.[10,35] The presence of VUE in pregnancies of mothers with inflammatory and autoimmune disorders, such as Behçet disease and neonatal alloimmune thrombocytopenia, also supports an immunologic origin[12,36] as well as the increased incidence of VUE in placentas from mothers with autoimmune disease.[13] Placentas from pregnancies with a donated ovum are a unique opportunity to study the placental response to an embryo in which neither embryonic haplotype matches that of the gestational carrier, making the embryo entirely an allograft as opposed to being the usual semiallograft. If the graft-versus-host hypothesis holds true, there should be an increased incidence and severity of VUE in the ovum-donated related placentas. Recent studies have shown there is at least twice the incidence of VUE in donor-ovum pregnancies, even compared with in vitro fertilization pregnancies using nondonor ovum. Fortunately, although there seems to be an increase in VUE in these pregnancies, the neonates produced from these donated ovum pregnancies are not at increased risk of adverse neonatal outcomes.[16,17] Although all these studies suggest that at least some incidences of VUE are caused by the maternal immune system not recognizing fetal antigen, they do not exclude the possibility that VUE is caused by maternal inflammatory cells recognizing a foreign antigen presented by fetal macrophages. VUE may also have a heterogeneous cause; because it is such a common lesion, one cause may not explain all occurrences.

CLINICAL OUTCOMES WITH VUE

Clinically, VUE is associated with premature delivery, IUGR, intrauterine fetal demise, neonatal neurologic impairment, and fetal death. In one study, VUE was the most common placental lesion associated with IUGR in normotensive pregnancy.[37] Not only the presence but also the grade of VUE is correlated with degree of IUGR. As severity of VUE increased, so did the incidence and severity of IUGR as well as incidence of perinatal mortality.[5] Mild or low-grade villitis, however, is not associated with poor neonatal outcome nor is it associated with the recurrence seen with more severe villitis.[5,6] It has long been recognized that there is a relationship between the VUE, increased maternal blood pressure, and IUGR.[2,9,11] VUE is specifically associated with preeclampsia as opposed to simply maternal hypertension and is found more often in preterm labor complicated by preeclampsia than spontaneous preterm labor.[15,38] VUE is also a risk factor for IUGR independent of maternal hypertension.[14] Severe VUE, when associated with fetal vascular thrombosis and obliteration, is associated with neonatal neurologic impairment and cerebral palsy.[6,39,40] It has been suggested that the combination of fetal vasculopathy and maternal inflammatory cells of VUE have a synergistic effect leading to increased fetal complications. Possible mechanisms include a systemic coagulopathy induced by the cytokines associated with VUE or direct damage to the fetus by the maternal lymphocytes.[39] Small case series have shown that recurrent VUE is associated with increased perinatal mortality.[35,41]

MASSIVE CHRONIC INTERVILLOSITIS

MCI, also known as chronic histiocytic intervillositis,[42] was first described in 1987 by Labarrere and Mullen.[43] This rare lesion, described as a fibrinoid and mononuclear infiltrate of the intervillous space, is often associated with VUE; however, the relationship has not been well defined. MCI also has no distinctive gross features.[44] Histologically, it is characterized by mononuclear cells, including lymphocytes, monocytes, and histiocytes, in the intervillous space (**Fig. 11**). Usually it is associated with

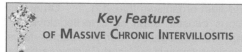

Key Features
OF MASSIVE CHRONIC INTERVILLOSITIS

Clinical
- History of MCI in the past
- Earlier presentation of MCI in recurrent cases

Gross Pathology
- No definitive gross lesion

Histology
- Histiocytes and fibrin in the intervillous space
- May be associated with VUE

variable amounts of fibrin deposition, although the presence of fibrin is not necessary to make the diagnosis.[1,42,44,45] Atherosis-like lesions in decidual vessels have also been described in MCI.[43]

DIAGNOSIS AND DIFFERENTIAL DIAGNOSIS OF MASSIVE CHRONIC INTERVILLOSITIS

The differential diagnosis of MCI is limited. Like VUE, MCI must also be distinguished from an intervillositis of infectious cause. The most well-documented infection associated with MCI is plasmodium infection, which can be confirmed by the presence of malaria pigment and

Fig. 11. Massive Chronic Intervillositis, (H&E, 10×).

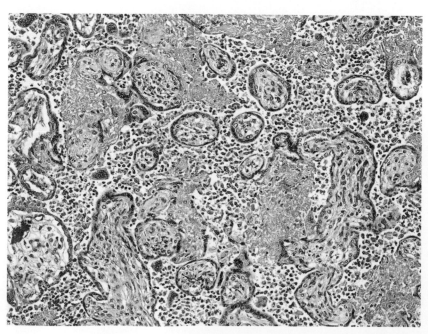

plasmodium organisms (**Fig. 12**).[46,47] Other rare infectious causes, such as cytomegalovirus,[48] *Listeria monocytogenes*, *Campylobacter fetus*, *Francisella tularensis*,[42,44] and *Chlamydia psittaci*,[49] have been reported. Again, a thorough clinical history can help differentiate between MCI and infectious intervillositis; however, there are few good histologic characteristics to distinguish the 2 entities, except for nuclear features specific to the infection, such as intracellular plasmodium or the owl-eye inclusion of CMV. The differential diagnosis of MCI also includes decidual necrosis and chronic deciduitis, perivillous fibrin deposition, maternal floor infarction, and diffuse VUE.

The pathology of MCI has not been well elucidated. It is often associated with VUE,[44,50] but that association is not necessary for diagnosis. Clinically, there has been some correlation with antiphospholipid syndrome.[44] Like VUE, MCI frequently recurs, often in greater severity during the recurrence, again implying an immunologic cause; however, there have been too few studies done to support any sort of hypothesis.

CLINICAL OUTCOMES WITH MCI

MCI is clinically associated with recurrent disease, poor fetal prognosis, and recurrent abortions. MCI has a high recurrence rate, reported at 80% to 100%, with recurrence often presenting earlier and earlier in gestational age.[35,41,42,51,52] The neonates that survive a pregnancy with MCI often have IUGR.[42,44] Rate of perinatal mortality associated with MCI has been reported to range from 29% to 83%.[42–44] Recurrent MCI is associated with a high spontaneous abortion rate, often with a normal fetal karyotype.[52,53] Although MCI has no symptoms, because of its high recurrence rate, there has been some suggestion that anti-inflammatory agents, such as prednisone, aspirin, and intravenous immunoglobulin, may be helpful in preventing spontaneous abortions in future pregnancies.[51]

ETIOLOGY OF MCI

VUE and MCI are both inflammatory lesions of the placenta that have unclear etiologies. VUE is a common lesion that may have no clinical consequence in its mildest form but in more severe grades is associated with poor neonatal outcome. MCI is a rare lesion; however, it is associated with a high recurrence rate that may lead to habitual abortions. These lesions must be differentiated from placental inflammation of an infectious etiology. This is most easily done with maternal clinical history, although there are some histologic clues that may help distinguish these entities. It is important to report the presence of these lesions in the diagnosis of a placenta because it may not only help explain the outcome of the current pregnancy but also help guide the clinical course in subsequent pregnancies.

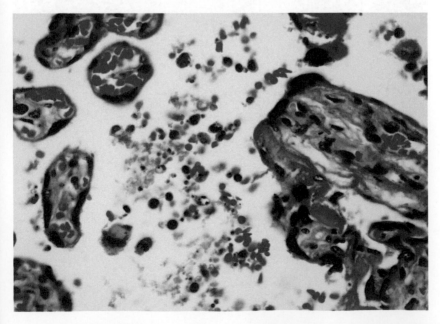

Fig. 12. Intraerythrocytic plasmodium and malarial pigment, (H&E, 40×).

REFERENCES

1. Benirschke K, Kaufmann P, Baergen R. Pathology of the human placenta. 5th edition. New York: Springer; 2006.
2. Knox WF, Fox H. Villitis of unknown aetiology: its incidence and significance in placentae from a British population. Placenta 1984;5(5):395–402.
3. Redline RW. Villitis of unknown etiology: noninfectious chronic villitis in the placenta. Hum Pathol 2007;38(10):1439–46.
4. Khong TY, Staples A, Moore L, et al. Observer reliability in assessing villitis of unknown aetiology. J Clin Pathol 1993;46(3):208–10.
5. Russell P. Inflammatory lesions of the human placenta. III: the histopathology of villitis of unknown aetiology. Placenta 1980;1:227–44.
6. Redline RW. Infections and other inflammatory conditions. Semin Diagn Pathol 2007;24(1):5–13.
7. Redline RW. Placental pathology: a systematic approach with clinical correlations. Placenta 2008; 29(Suppl A):S86–91.
8. Redline RW, Ariel I, Baergen RN, et al. Fetal vascular obstructive lesions: nosology and reproducibility of placental reaction patterns. Pediatr Dev Pathol 2004;7(5):443–52.
9. Althabe O, Labarrere C. Chronic villitis of unknown aetiology and intrauterine growth-retarded infants of normal and low ponderal index. Placenta 1985; 6(4):369–73.
10. Labarrere C, Althabe O. Chronic villitis of unknown aetiology in recurrent intrauterine fetal growth retardation. Placenta 1987;8(2):167–73.
11. Labarrere C, Althabe O, Telenta M. Chronic villitis of unknown aetiology in placentae of idiopathic small for gestational age infants. Placenta 1982;3(3): 309–17.
12. Althaus J, Weir EG, Askin F, et al. Chronic villitis in untreated neonatal alloimmune thrombocytopenia: an etiology for severe early intrauterine growth restriction and the effect of intravenous immunoglobulin therapy. Am J Obstet Gynecol 2005;193(3 Pt 2): 1100–4.
13. Labarrere CA, et al. Placental lesions in maternal autoimmune diseases. Am J Reprod Immunol Microbiol 1986;12(3):78–86.
14. Labarrere C, Althabe O. Chronic villitis of unknown etiology and maternal arterial lesions in preeclamptic pregnancies. Eur J Obstet Gynecol Reprod Biol 1985;20(1):1–11.
15. Labarrere C, Althabe O. Chronic villitis of unknown aetiology and decidual maternal vasculopathies in sustained chronic hypertension. Eur J Obstet Gynecol Reprod Biol 1986;21(1):27–32.
16. Perni SC, Predanic M, Cho JE, et al. Placental pathology and pregnancy outcomes in donor and non-donor oocyte in vitro fertilization pregnancies. J Perinat Med 2005;33(1):27–32.
17. Styer AK, et al. Placental villitis of unclear etiology during ovum donor in vitro fertilization pregnancy. Am J Obstet Gynecol 2003;189(4):1184–6.
18. Feeley L, Mooney EE. Villitis of unknown aetiology: correlation of recurrence with clinical outcome. J Obstet Gynaecol 2010;30(5):476–9.
19. Baergen RN. Manual of pathology of the human placenta. 2nd edition. New York: Springer; 2011.
20. Abramowsky CR, Gutman J, Hilinski J. Mycobacterium tuberculosis infection of the placenta: a study of the early (innate) inflammatory response in two cases. Pediatr Dev Pathol 2012;15(2):132–6.
21. Jezova M, Muckova K, Koukalova P. Spontaneus abortion caused by Listeria monocytogenes–report of three cases. Cesk Patol 2008;44(3):71–4 [in Czech].
22. Sheikh SS, Amr SS, Lage JM. Acute placental infection due to Klebsiella pneumoniae: report of a unique case. Infect Dis Obstet Gynecol 2005;13(1):49–52.
23. Petignat P, Vial Y, Laurini R, et al. Fetal varicella-herpes zoster syndrome in early pregnancy: ultrasonographic and morphological correlation. Prenat Diagn 2001;21(2):121–4.
24. Altemani AM, Bittencourt AL, Lana AM. Immunohistochemical characterization of the inflammatory infiltrate in placental Chagas' disease: a qualitative and quantitative analysis. Am J Trop Med Hyg 2000; 62(2):319–24.
25. Syridou G, Spanakis N, Konstandinou A, et al. Detection of cytomegalovirus, parvovirus B19 and herpes simplex viruses in cases of intrauterine fetal death: association with pathological findings. J Med Virol 2008;80(10):1776–82.
26. Rivasi F, Gasser B, Bagni A, et al. Placental candidiasis: report of four cases, one with villitis. APMIS 1998;106(12):1165–9.
27. Altemani A, Gonzatti A, Metze K. How many paraffin blocks are necessary to detect villitis? Placenta 2003;24(1):116–7.
28. Brito H, Juliano P, Altemani C, et al. Is the immunohistochemical study of the inflammatory infiltrate helpful in distinguishing villitis of unknown etiology from non-specific infection villitis? Placenta 2005; 26(10):839–41.
29. Ernst LM, Crouch J, Rinder H, et al. Bacterial etiology for chronic villitis is not supported by polymerase chain reaction for 16S rRNA DNA. Pediatr Dev Pathol 2005;8(6):647–53.
30. Kim MJ, Romero R, Kim CJ, et al. Villitis of unknown etiology is associated with a distinct pattern of chemokine up-regulation in the feto-maternal and placental compartments: implications for conjoint maternal allograft rejection and maternal anti-fetal graft-versus-host disease. J Immunol 2009;182(6): 3919–27.

31. Labarrere CA, Faulk WP. Maternal cells in chorionic villi from placentae of normal and abnormal human pregnancies. Am J Reprod Immunol 1995;33(1): 54–9.

32. Redline RW, Patterson P. Villitis of unknown etiology is associated with major infiltration of fetal tissue by maternal inflammatory cells. Am J Pathol 1993; 143(2):473–9.

33. Kim JS, Romero R, Kim MR, et al. Involvement of Hofbauer cells and maternal T cells in villitis of unknown aetiology. Histopathology 2008;52(4):457–64.

34. Myerson D, Parkin RK, Bernischke K, et al. The pathogenesis of villitis of unknown etiology: analysis with a new conjoint immunohistochemistry-in situ hybridization procedure to identify specific maternal and fetal cells. Pediatr Dev Pathol 2006;9(4):257–65.

35. Redline RW, Abramowsky CR. Clinical and pathologic aspects of recurrent placental villitis. Hum Pathol 1985;16(7):727–31.

36. Hwang I, Lee CK, Yoo B, et al. Necrotizing villitis and decidual vasculitis in the placentas of mothers with Behcet disease. Hum Pathol 2009;40(1):135–8.

37. Redline RW, Patterson P. Patterns of placental injury. Correlations with gestational age, placental weight, and clinical diagnoses. Arch Pathol Lab Med 1994; 118(7):698–701.

38. Salafia CM, Pezzullo JC, Lopez-Zeno JA, et al. Placental pathologic features of preterm preeclampsia. Am J Obstet Gynecol 1995;173(4): 1097–105.

39. Redline RW. Severe fetal placental vascular lesions in term infants with neurologic impairment. Am J Obstet Gynecol 2005;192(2):452–7.

40. McDonald DG, et al. Placental fetal thrombotic vasculopathy is associated with neonatal encephalopathy. Hum Pathol 2004;35(7):875–80.

41. Russell P, Atkinson K, Krishnan L. Recurrent reproductive failure due to severe placental villitis of unknown etiology. J Reprod Med 1980;24(2):93–8.

42. Boyd TK, Redline RW. Chronic histiocytic intervillositis: a placental lesion associated with recurrent reproductive loss. Hum Pathol 2000;31(11):1389–96.

43. Labarrere C, Mullen E. Fibrinoid and trophoblastic necrosis with massive chronic intervillositis: an extreme variant of villitis of unknown etiology. Am J Reprod Immunol Microbiol 1987;15(3):85–91.

44. Parant O, Capdet J, Kessler S, et al. Chronic intervillositis of unknown etiology (CIUE): relation between placental lesions and perinatal outcome. Eur J Obstet Gynecol Reprod Biol 2009;143(1):9–13.

45. Marchaudon V, Devisme L, Petit S, et al. Chronic histiocytic intervillositis of unknown etiology: clinical features in a consecutive series of 69 cases. Placenta 2011;32(2):140–5.

46. Nebuloni M, Pallotti F, Polizzotti G, et al. Malaria placental infection with massive chronic intervillositis in a gravida 4 woman. Hum Pathol 2001;32(9): 1022–3.

47. Ordi J, Ismail MR, Ventura PJ, et al. Massive chronic intervillositis of the placenta associated with malaria infection. Am J Surg Pathol 1998;22(8):1006–11.

48. Taweevisit M, Sukpan K, Siriaunkqui S, et al. Chronic histiocytic intervillositis with cytomegalovirus placentitis in a case of hydrops fetalis. Fetal Pediatr Pathol 2012;31(6):394–400.

49. Hyde SR, Benirschke K. Gestational psittacosis: case report and literature review. Mod Pathol 1997; 10(6):602–7.

50. Rota C, Carles D, Schaeffer V, et al. Perinatal prognosis of pregnancies complicated by placental chronic intervillitis. J Gynecol Obstet Biol Reprod (Paris) 2006;35(7):711–9 [in French].

51. Boog G, Le Vaillant C, Alnoukari F, et al. Combining corticosteroid and aspirin for the prevention of recurrent villitis or intervillositis of unknown etiology. J Gynecol Obstet Biol Reprod (Paris) 2006;35(4): 396–404 [in French].

52. Doss BJ, Greene MF, Hill J, et al. Massive chronic intervillositis associated with recurrent abortions. Hum Pathol 1995;26(11):1245–51.

53. Salafia C, Maier D, Vogel C, et al. Placental and decidual histology in spontaneous abortion: detailed description and correlations with chromosome number. Obstet Gynecol 1993;82(2):295–303.

Placental Mesenchymal Dysplasia

Ona Marie Faye-Petersen, MD[a,b,*], Raj P. Kapur, MD, PhD[c]

KEYWORDS

- Placental mesenchymal dysplasia • Partial mole • Pseudo-partial mole
- Androgenetic-biparental mosaicism • Placental mosaicism • Mesenchymal hamartoma • Imprinting
- Chorangiomatosis

ABSTRACT

Placental mesenchymal dysplasia is a rare, incompletely understood placental stromal lesion, characterized by placentomegaly and striking ectasia and tortuosity of chorionic plate and stem villous vessels. Its prenatal ultrasonographic and gross pathologic features resemble those of a partial mole, but the fetus is typically normal and the placenta has a diploid, chromosomal complement. We discuss the pathologic features and current understanding of the etiopathogenesis of this condition, the supportive immunohistochemical and confirmatory molecular genetic studies important in its diagnosis, and its implications for pregnancy and infant outcomes.

OVERVIEW

Placental mesenchymal dysplasia (PMD) is an incompletely understood, rare anomaly (0.02% estimated incidence)[1] with a strong female predominance (3.6–4.0: 1)[2,3] seen among the approximately 90 cases reported during the past 2 decades.[1–36] PMD is characterized by placentomegaly, cirsoid vessels of the chorionic plate and stem villi, and grapelike villous vesicles, and has been referred to as "pseudo-partial" or "partly partial" mole[2,4–6]; however, the fetus is often structurally normal. Prenatal ultrasonography of PMD reveals an enlarged, thickened placenta with hyperechoic (cystic) areas concentrated in the

Key Points
PLACENTAL MESENCHYMAL DYSPLASIA

- Rare, sporadic lesion also known as "pseudo-partial mole," "pseudo-mole," and "partly partial mole"; however, karyotype is diploid, and fetus is often structurally normal and female (F:M ratio ~4:1)

- Placentomegaly, foci of vascular ectasia, and tortuosity in chorionic plate and stem villi, stromal cisterns, and scattered hydropic grapelike villi admixed with normal villi

- Trophoblastic hyperplasia and pseudoinclusions *not* present

- Incompletely understood pathogenesis, but most cases have immunohistochemical and/or molecular genetic evidence of chorionic mesenchymal stromal mosaicism in abnormal villi:

  o Abnormally vascularized, edematous and cistern-containing villi, although diploid, show abnormal presence of cells with evidence of paternal uniparental disomy (diploid, but all alleles are paternally derived) and/or loss of maternal imprinting at specific loci

  o Normal villi display normal, biparental diploid genetic complement

- Fetal associations: intrauterine growth restriction (common), Beckwith-Wiedemann Syndrome, fetal/neonatal mesenchymal hamartomas of viscera and skin, autosomal recessive disorder in fetus wherein father is the only parent carrier

- High perinatal morbidity and mortality rates

[a] Pathology, The University of Alabama at Birmingham, 619 19th Street South, NP 3547, Birmingham, AL 35249-7331, USA; [b] Obstetrics and Gynecology, The University of Alabama at Birmingham, 619 19th Street South, NP 3547, Birmingham, AL 35249-7331, USA; [c] Department of Laboratories, The University of Washington, Seattle Children's Hospital & Regional Medical Center, A6901, 4800 Sand Point Way, NE, Seattle, WA 98105, USA
* Corresponding author. Pathology, The University of Alabama at Birmingham, 619 19th Street South, NP 3547, Birmingham, AL 35249-7331.
E-mail address: onafp@uab.edu

Surgical Pathology 6 (2013) 127–151
http://dx.doi.org/10.1016/j.path.2012.11.007

subchorionic zone. Although cystic changes may be seen at 8 weeks,[1] they are typically detected in the second trimester[31] and progressively enlarge, becoming more numerous and complex as gestation proceeds.[1,11] Pathologic correlations of these progressions are evident when midgestational placentas with PMD are compared with those from third-trimester deliveries. The vascular abnormalities of PMD lead to chorionic villous dysfunction, edematous distension, thrombosis, and fetal intrauterine growth restriction (IUGR), and/or perinatal demise.

The diagnosis of PMD is best supported by detection of confined placental androgenetic/biparental mosaicism (ABM)[5,6,16,17,21,24,37–40] and/or allelic imbalance of imprinted genes,[4,7,11,13,17,24,28,41] and similar imbalance may occasionally affect fetal tissues.[2,12,21,23,26,32,35,42]

GROSS FEATURES OF PMD

Generally, the placenta with PMD is enlarged for gestational dates, in dimension and weight, but

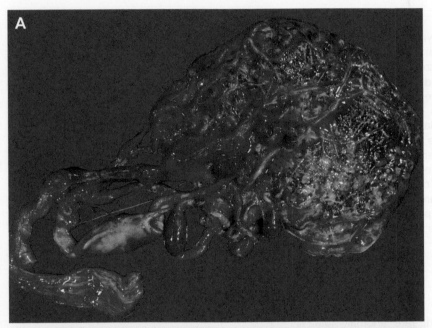

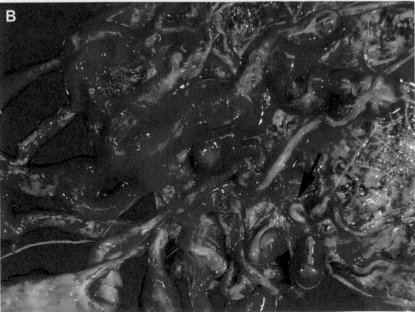

Fig. 1. Gross characteristic features of PMD. (*A*) PMD is typified by placentomegaly and the presence of ectatic to bulbous-appearing, tortuous, thick-walled vessels on chorionic plate, as seen on this specimen. (*B*) Closer inspection of the entanglement of vessels shows that both arterial and venous chorionic vessels (arteries cross over veins on the fetal surface) are dysplastic with aneursymal dilatations and patchy thrombosis (*arrow*). (Thrombi may be grossly identified, on the *fresh* specimen, by gentle pressure on the vessels, because blood will not move passively past an obstruction.) (*Courtesy of* R.D. LeGallo, MD, Department of Pathology, University of Virginia, Charlottesville, VA.)

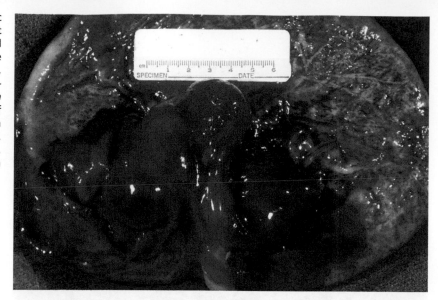

Fig. 2. Gross chorionic plate from a different case of PMD. Large, dilated and redundant vessels are surrounded by viscous, edematous connective tissue and blood. (*From* Baergen RN. Manual of pathology of the human placenta. 2nd edition. New York: Springer; 2011. p. 372, Fig. 19.18; with permission.)

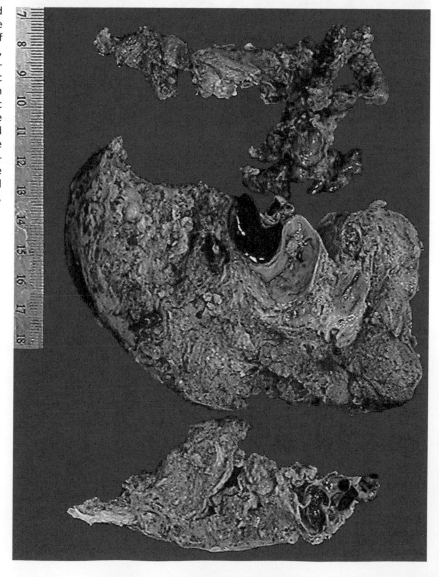

Fig. 3. Fixed sectioned specimen with PMD. The umbilical cord is a mass of redundant ectactic vessels, and sections show massively dilated subchorionic vessels. The bottom section shows that the cystic structures extend to the paramarginal regions, and deeply, to approximate the maternal surface. (*Courtesy of* D.S. Heller, MD, the University of Medicine and Dentistry of New Jersey, Newark, NJ.)

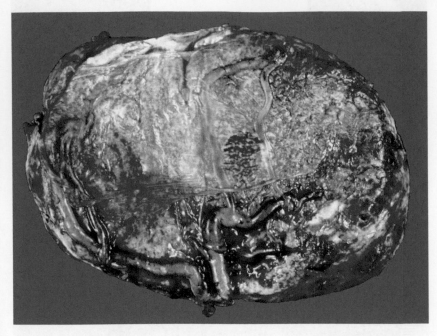

Fig. 4. Placenta from delivery of live-born infant with Beckwith-Wiedemann syndrome at 36 weeks of gestation. This placenta was 1050 g (372–542 g expected.) The trivascular umbilical cord had a marginal insertion (not shown), but was submitted as a separate, 90-cm-long segment that demonstrated numerous varices and excessive coiling. The chorionic plate of the placenta shows markedly ectatic and abnormally branching arteries and veins with intervening, abnormal net-like patterns of ramifications. The parenchyma was 3.5 cm thick with numerous cystic foci.

the hallmark is the presence of ectatic to bulbous-appearing, tortuous, thick-walled vessels, on the chorionic plate, and umbilical cord varices.[1,2,4–16] The chorionic dysplastic vessels are frequently bordered by gelatinous substance, and, sometimes, by extravasated chorionic blood or clot (**Figs. 1–4**).[1,2] Thrombosis is common. As noted, PMD is associated with Beckwith-Wiedemann Syndrome (BWS) (see **Fig. 4**), and, in these instances, excessive cord length, hypercoiling, and/or varix formation is particularly common; however, placentomegaly and insertional, umbilical arterial, and cord-coiling abnormalities also occur in PMD cases without BWS.[2] The maternal surface shows patchy distribution of hydropic villi in a background of normal-appearing villous tissue (**Fig. 5**). These latter findings are suggestive of a partial mole,[1,2,4–6] but, in PMD, the large cystlike

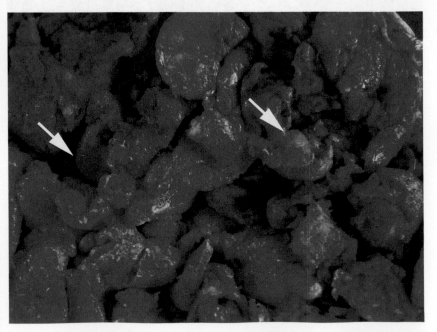

Fig. 5. Maternal surface from markedly enlarged placenta with gross and histologic morphology of PMD. Arrows show pedunculated, cystic villi interspersed among grossly normal villous tissue; the gross features were suggestive of a partial hydatidiform mole.

Fig. 6. Cut surfaces of placenta in **Fig. 5** (*A, B*). Sections show numerous, small grapelike cysts in the parenchyma of this case of PMD, that ranged from 0.2 to 1.2 cm in diameter (*arrows* in *A* show examples). (*B*) This image shows an opened cyst from the maternal surface demonstrated in **Fig. 5**, and reveals its continuity with villous vascular branches. (*C*) This image shows ropey, thickened, villous branch vessels, in a gelatinous connective tissue, nearly extending to the maternal surface.

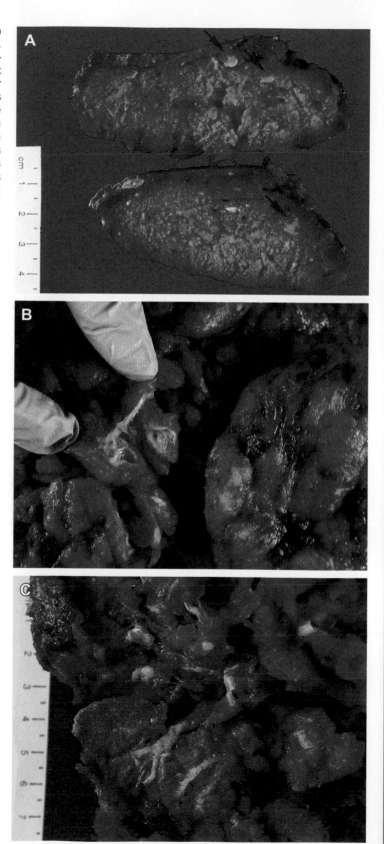

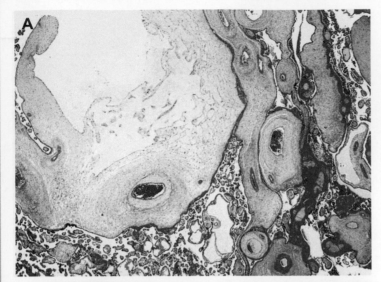

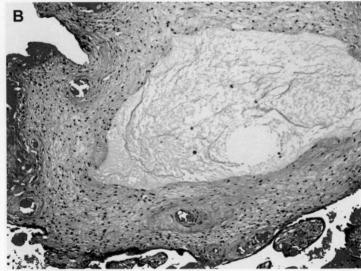

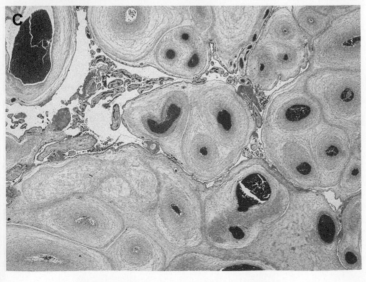

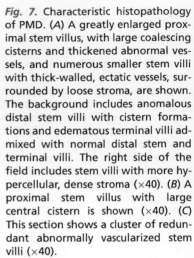

Fig. 7. Characteristic histopathology of PMD. (*A*) A greatly enlarged proximal stem villus, with large coalescing cisterns and thickened abnormal vessels, and numerous smaller stem villi with thick-walled, ectatic vessels, surrounded by loose stroma, are shown. The background includes anomalous distal stem villi with cistern formations and edematous terminal villi admixed with normal distal stem and terminal villi. The right side of the field includes stem villi with more hypercellular, dense stroma (×40). (*B*) A proximal stem villus with large central cistern is shown (×40). (*C*) This section shows a cluster of redundant abnormally vascularized stem villi (×40).

Fig. 7. (*D*) This image shows a stem villus with central myxomatous stroma and peripheral distribution of thick-walled vessels, in a mixed background of small normal and dysmature villi (×40). (*E*) A distal stem villous shows cistern formations and thick-walled vessels in a field of normal and edematous terminal villi (×100). ([*A, E*] *Courtesy of* R.D. LeGallo, MD, Department of Pathology, University of Virginia, Charlottesville, VA.)

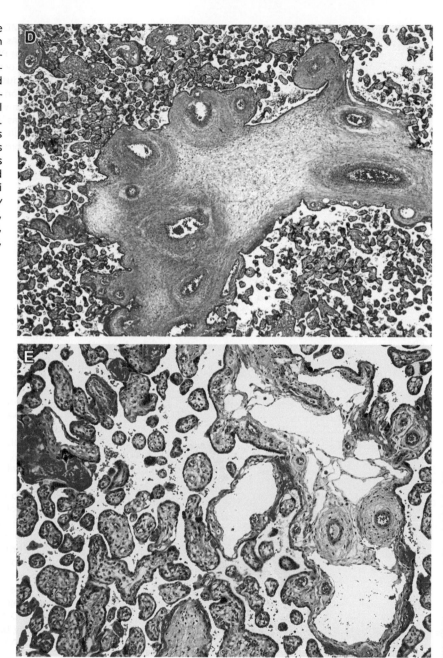

structures, particularly those in the subchorionic zone, are predominantly aneursymally dilated *vessels* in an edematous, loose connective tissue. Serial sections typically reveal tortuous, myxomatous stem villi and scattered, "grapelike" villous vesicles containing colorless and thin to cloudy and mucinous fluid (see **Fig. 2**; **Fig. 6**). Complex cirsoid vessels and hydropic villi are more evident in placentas from more advanced gestations, and are likely pathologic correlates of the progressive, ultrasonographic findings of PMD. They suggest that the vascular malformations of PMD undergo progressive dysplasia/hyperplasia, which results in vascular redundancy, luminal pressure changes, and ectasias.

MICROSCOPIC FEATURES OF PMD

PMD is best appreciated at low power (×20), as the groups of abnormal villi are interspersed with normal-appearing villi. The affected proximal stem villi are bulky, with moderately to markedly

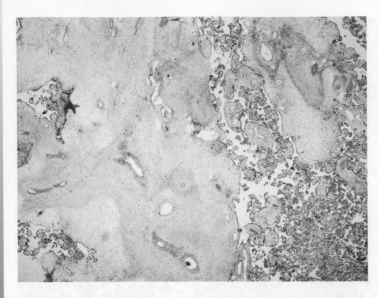

Fig. 8. PMD with fibromatous villous stroma. As in **Fig. 7**, the histopathology of PMD may include the findings of occasional stem villi with fibromatous stroma and few to no cistern formations. The large and ramifying villus on the left, in this image, has some myxomatous areas, but its bulk is primarily because of its dense, fibromatous stroma (×20).

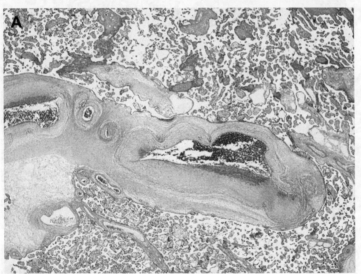

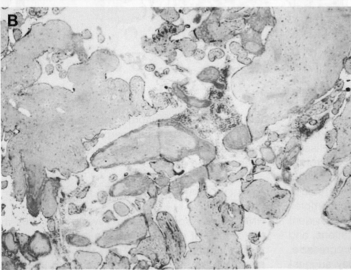

Fig. 9. PMD complicated by fetal thrombotic vasculopathy (FTV). (*A*) Ectatic, tortuous, myxomatous vessels within a large-stem villus from a case of PMD shows acute mural thrombi. The background shows edematous villi with myxomatous stroma and cisterns admixed with more normal-appearing chorionic villi (×20). (*B*) Clusters of sclerotic, involuted distal and terminal chorionic villi are present. A few viable terminal villi are seen in the upper right corner of the field. Other features of PMD, also seen in **Fig. 8**, include the presence of thick, bulky stem and distal villi with fibromatous stroma and abnormal patterns of vascularization (×40). Thrombi may contribute to abnormal blood flow patterns and pressures in the remaining chorionic villous tree and further contribute to the chorionic villous maldevelopment in PMD. (*Courtesy of* R.D. LeGallo, MD, Department of Pathology, University of Virginia, Charlottesville, VA.)

Fig. 10. Composite of various coexistent villous capillary lesions that may be seen in PMD. (*A*) *Chorangiosis* (defined as the presence of 10 or more capillary outlines in 10 or more terminal villi evaluated with a ×10 objective, in 3 different, noninfarcted, chorionic villous fields) is present in this representative field from a case of PMD. Scattered, sclerotic terminal villi (FTV) are also seen (×100 original total magnification). (*B*) A microscopic *chorangioma*, composed of a well- demarcated, rounded mass of numerous capillaries covered by trophoblast, is shown (×40). (*C*) This gross image of a massive, bulging chorangioma shows its vascular supply on the chorionic plate.

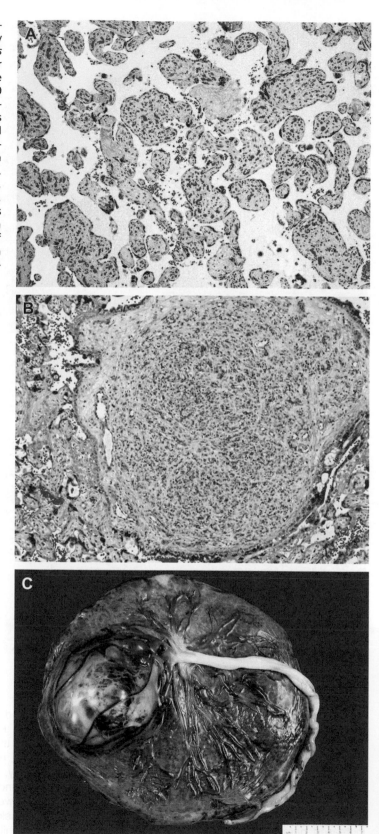

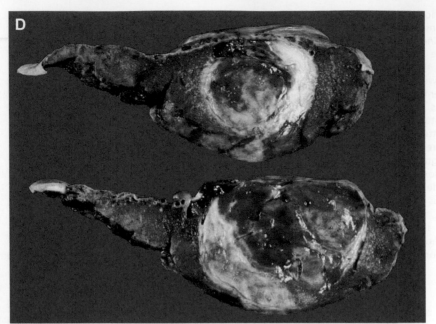

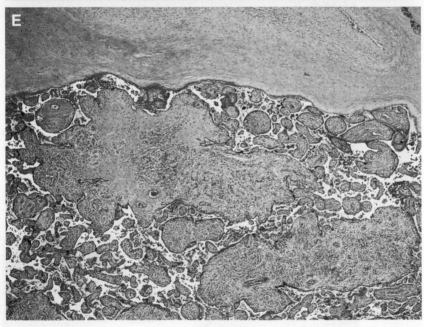

Fig. 10. (*D*) The cut surfaces of the lesion in (*C*) reveal a circumscribed mass of firm tissue with areas of hemorrhage and infarction. (*E, F*) *Chorangiomatosis* is a multifocal, capillary proliferative and permeative lesion that involves otherwise normal distal branch stem and immature intermediate villi, as depicted here (*E*, ×40; *F*, ×100).

ectatic, thick-walled vessels and loose, connective tissue with cistern formations. The cisterns contain amphophilic to faintly eosinophilic fluid, and may be large and coalescing, or multiple, irregular, fragile-appearing, fluid pockets (**Fig. 7**A, B). Microscopic sections show clusters of anomalous stem villi with thickened vessels (see **Fig. 7**C). Distal branches of the villous tree generally exhibit increased numbers of peripherally located, predominantly thick-walled, disproportionately small vessels and central cistern formations (see **Fig. 7**D, E). Hydropic, distal villi may be so distended that their vessels are difficult to identify or "absent" (ie, hydropic degeneration) (see **Fig. 7**E). Occasionally, stem villi show a central myxoid axis surrounded by more fibromatous stroma (**Fig. 8**); however, trophoblastic proliferation and pseudoinclusions are not present and villous surfaces exhibit a simple, trophoblastic epithelial covering. The abnormal chorionic plate and stem

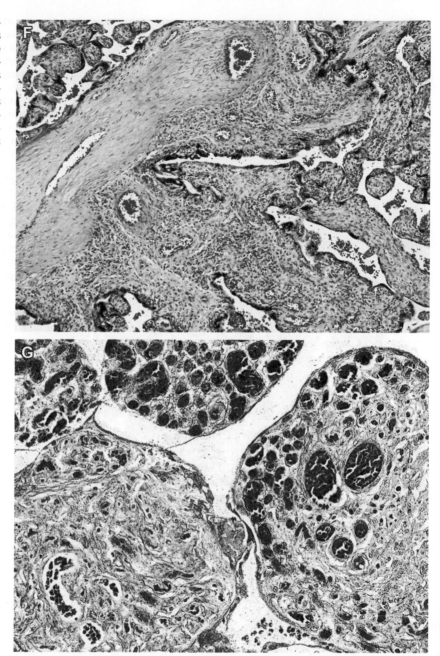

Fig. 10. (G) The numerous of small capillaries of chorangiomatosis are surrounded by a continuous layer of pericytes and imbedded in a reticulin fiber-rich stroma, as evidenced by the histochemical staining for reticulin fibers in this image (×400).

villous vessels, probably because of their tortuosity and secondary aberrations in fetal blood flow dynamics, commonly show asymmetric, mural attenuation and a full spectrum of fetal thrombotic vasculopathic lesions (FTVs) including nonocclusive to occlusive, acute, chronic, or propagating thrombi (see the article by F. Kraus elsewhere in this issue) (**Fig. 9**A). Distal villi may also show vascular, aneursymal dilatations and thromboses,

coupled with chorionic villous degenerative FTVs, including erythrocyte extravasation, stromal karyorrhexis, and sclerosis (see **Fig. 9**B).[1,2,4–16] The histopathology of PMD may include foci of chorangiosis (**Fig. 10**A), chorangioma (see **Fig. 10**B), and chorangiomatosis (see **Fig. 10**E–G).[2,3,22,43–46] Increased numbers of circulating fetal nucleated red blood cells (NRBCs) or normoblastemia, are not uncommon. Frank erythroblastosis (**Fig. 11**A)

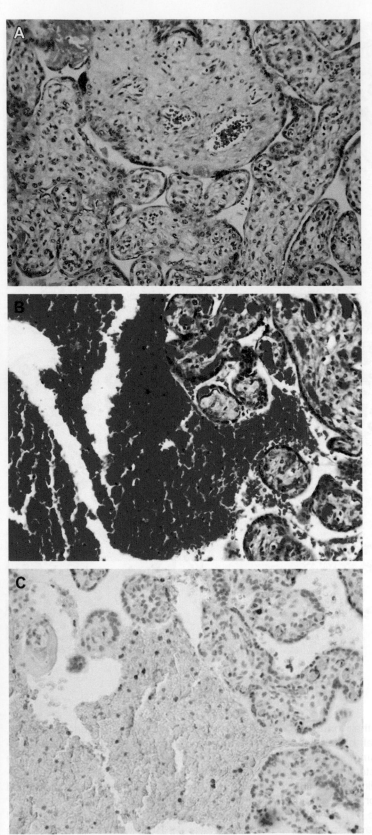

Fig. 11. PMD complicated by fetal erythroblastosis and fetomaternal hemorrhage (documented fetal anemia and positive maternal Kleihauer-Betke test). (*A*) Chorionic villi show capillaries containing numerous NRBCs, including larger, more immature pronormoblast forms (×400). (*B*) NRBCs are seen in the maternal space; their numbers are far in excess of normal numbers of circulating NRBCs in adult peripheral blood (×200). (*C*) The immunohistochemical stain for fetal hemoglobin (performed at Nationwide Children's Hospital Pathology Laboratory, Columbus, OH) shows cytoplasmic staining of nucleated and non-nucleated erythrocytes in the maternal space and in the villous capillaries. Thus, the number of NRBCs in the perivillous space detectable by hematoxylin-eosin stain is a small fraction of the total number of fetal RBCs present (×200).

PMD	Differential Entity
1. Enlarged, abnormally vascularized chorionic villi with variably cellular stroma, large cistern formations; numerous stromal vessels positioned peripherally in distal chorionic villous branches; thrombi common	*Partial Hydatidiform Mole*[2,5,47–50] 1. Vascularized, but edematous, enlarged, immature-appearing villi, with scarce microcistern formations; vessels may show ectasia, but do not exhibit mural thickening or thrombi
2. No trophoblastic proliferation	2. Lacelike, scalloped, trophoblastic proliferations and pseudoinclusions
3. Chorionic plate and proximal stem villous vascular ectasia and redundancy, with generally thickened, myxomatous walls	3. Edema and cistern formations spare proximal stem villi; focal stromal fibrosis may be seen
4. Fields of malformed villi are interspersed with normal villi	4. Dimorphic population of hydropic villi and intervening normal-appearing villi
5. Diploid karyotype (~80% 46,XX; ~20% 46,XY): androgenetic/biparental mosaicism identified in most cases	5. Triploid placenta and fetus: triploidy usually due to dispermic fertilization of single ovum (diandric conceptus); most common karyotype 69,XXY
6. Fetus often structurally normal, but growth restricted	6. Anomalous fetus: severe IUGR with hydrocephaly, third to fourth digital syndactyly, midline facial clefting, and cardiovascular and renal anomalies
7. Associated with BWS in one-fourth to one-third of cases	
As above	*Complete Hydatidiform Mole*[2,5,47–50] 1. Diffusely distributed, large, avascular, hydropic villi with large central cisterns surrounded by loose, hypocellular stroma
	2. Abundant, often circumferential (nonpolar) cyto- trophoblastic and syncytio-trophoblastic proliferation
	3. Trophoblastic atypia and mitoses present with nuclear pleomorphism and cyto-trophoblastic and syncytio-trophoblastic vacuoles
	4. Diploid karyotype: in second-trimester and third-trimester cases, diploidy most often reflects diandric origin of conceptus
	5. Embryo/fetus *rarely* present
1. Coexistent chorangiomas are microscopic or very small	*Multiple chorangiomas*[2,43] 1. Bulging, well-circumscribed, usually paramarginally located, hamartomatous masses with vascular supply typically identifiable on fetal surface
	2. Microscopic appearance of central expansion of stem villus, by myriad capillaries in scant stroma, covered by trophoblast
	3. Does not exhibit aneursymally dilated, tortuous, large vessels

1. Chorionic vessels cystically dilated and ectatic and may show perivascular hemorrhage and hemosiderin-laden macrophages in chorionic stroma, and cisterns may be massive, but no true cysts with epithelial lining

2. Anomalous, cirsoid vascular and villous stromal elements affect chorion, and primary, proximal, and branching parenchymal, distal villi; cystic dilatations largest in, but not isolated to, chorion and subchorionic region

Multiple massive subchorionic cysts and/or cystic thrombohematomas

1. Large to massive cysts lined by extravillous cytotrophoblast, filled with thin proteinaceous, amphophilic fluid

2. Chorionic vessels and chorioamnion attenuated and splayed over cysts' surfaces, but otherwise structurally normal

3. Maternal blood contamination of cystic contents evidenced as extravasated, degenerating erythrocytes in fluid and/or cyst lining or hemosiderin deposition

4. Large subchorionic thrombohematomas with degenerative change may leak into or contribute to formation of subchorionic cyst

5. Location of cysts and thrombohematomas limited to subchorionic region

---

1. Affects umbilical cord, chorionic plate, and proximal stem villi, as well as distal stem villi

2. Villous stroma may be hypercellular, but pericytes not present and reticulin scant

3. Coexistent chorangiomatosis is scattered finding, not predominant histopathology

Multifocal chorangiomatosis[43]

1. Villous capillary lesion of immature distal branch stem or immature intermediate villi; not lesion of chorionic plate or proximal villi

2. Villi have numerous, small, thin-walled vessels surrounded by pericytes and dense stromal reticulin

---

and the presence of excessive numbers of NRBCs, in the perivillous space, may be seen in cases of PMD complicated by fetomaternal hemorrhage (FMH)[33] (O.M.F.-P. observation) (see **Fig. 11**B, C).

DIFFERENTIAL DIAGNOSIS OF PMD

PMD must be distinguished clinically and pathologically from partial hydatidiform mole, complete hydatidiform mole, multiple chorangiomas, and multiple, large subchorionic cysts and/or cystic thrombohematomas. The pathologic differential also includes diffuse multifocal chorangiomatosis and fetoplacental hydrops caused by chronic fetomaternal hemorrhage.

A full description of the pathology of gestational trophoblastic disease[47–50] is beyond the scope of this discussion, but partial hydaditiform mole has hydropic, vascularized villi and can occasionally exhibit dilated, central vessels. Partial molar placental villi show significant trophoblastic proliferation and pseudoinclusions (**Fig. 12**) and a triploid karyotype, however, and the corresponding fetus has multiple anomalies. The complete hydatidiform mole is diploid, but has diffuse, massively hydropic, *avascular* villi with abundant, trophoblastic proliferation (**Fig. 13**).

Chorangiomas[2,43,44] are bulging villous hamartomas that typically arise from stem villi close to the fetal surface, and show prominent "feeder vessels" (see **Fig. 10**C, D). Microscopically, they are well-circumscribed masses of small capillaries embedded in scant connective tissue and covered by trophoblast (see **Fig. 10**B). Although their appearance suggests a centrally expanded stem villus, myxoid variants exist, and degenerative features (thrombosis, infarction, hemorrhage, calcification) are common (see **Fig. 10**D); the spectrum and distribution of the aneurysmally dilated, convoluted vessels of PMD are not seen.

Diffuse, multifocal chorangiomatosis, the type of chorangiomatosis (vs localized focal and segmental forms) more likely to be confused with PMD, does not affect umbilical cord or chorionic plate vessels, or produce cirsoid, cavernous vessels in the plate, or ectatic vessels in primary stem villi. Multifocal chorangiomatosis is a villous capillary lesion that affects immature, more distal branch stem or immature intermediate villi. The vessels in chorangiomatosis are small, numerous, typically do not have thickened walls, are surrounded by alpha–smooth muscle actin–positive pericytes, and are distributed in a dense reticulin fiber-rich stroma (see **Fig. 10**E–G).[43,46] As noted

Fig. 12. Histopathology of partial hydatidiform mole. (*A*) Chorionic villi are vascularized but exhibit edema, with small cistern formations, peripheral scalloping, and mild trophoblastic proliferation with a lacelike pattern (×40). (*B*) Other fields reveal that there is a dimorphic population with nonmolar and molar villi, with some showing villous sclerosis (×40).

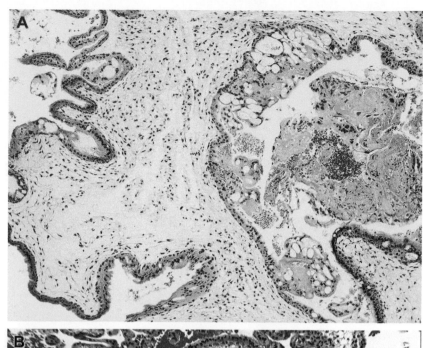

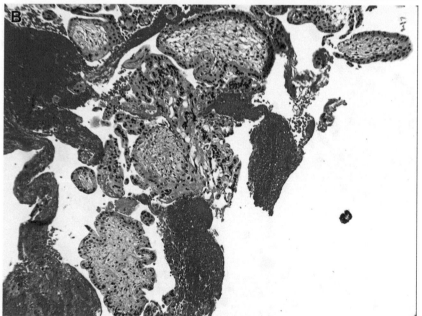

previously, because hypoxic stimulus contributes to the development of chorangiosis, and may contribute to the vascular proliferations in chorangioma and/or chorangiomatosis,[2,43,45] these other villous capillary lesions may coexist in some cases of PMD.

Subchorionic cysts, up to a few centimeters in diameter, contain clear serous or mucinlike proteinaceous fluid, and are found in 5% to 7% of mature placentas.[2] Rarely, *multiple*, large and bulging cysts may develop, and these, in the authors' experience, have been confused with PMD in prenatal ultrasonograms (**Fig. 14**A). The cysts, which are lined by extravillous trophoblast cells that elaborate major basic and other proteins, push the overlying and secondarily thinned chorioamnion upward, and show central liquefaction of degenerated trophoblasts and their matrix material (see **Fig. 14**B, C). Cystic degeneration may include "contamination" of the cyst contents

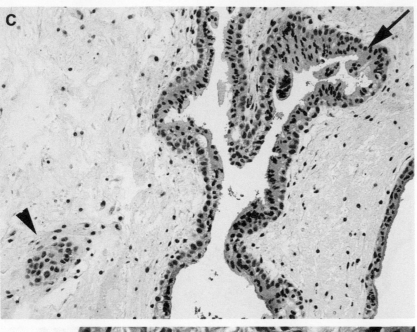

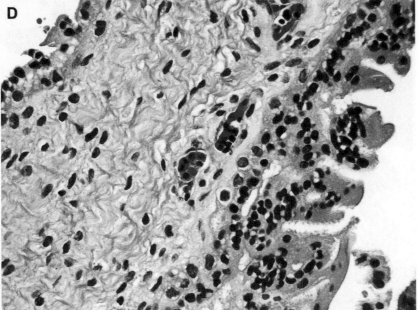

Fig. 12. (*C*) Higher magnification shows invaginations (*arrow*) result in pseudoinclusions (*arrowhead*) (×100). (*D*) Villous capillaries contain fetal nucleated erythrocytes (×400). ([*B, D*] *From* Heller DS. Gestational trophoblastic disease. In: McManus LW, Mitchell RN, editors. Pathobiology of human disease: a dynamic encyclopedia of disease mechanisms. Philadelphia: Elsevier; in press.)

by blood from the underlying maternal space, and grossly result in a brownish to greenish-yellow fluid tinge (see **Fig. 14**A) and hemosiderin deposition, microscopically. However, subchorionic cysts may represent degeneration of chronic subchorionic thrombohematomas (ie, large accumulations of maternal blood admixed with layered fibrin underlying the chorionic plate) (see **Fig. 14**D), which displace villi laterally, and which

protrude from the fetal surface (so-called Breus moles). The latter are associated with maternal thrombophilias[51] and preeclampsia and adverse perinatal outcomes,[52] but chorionic plate, stem, and distal chorionic villous vessels are not ectatic, tortuous, or dysplastic, and stem villi are structurally normal.

Fetoplacental hydrops, secondary to chronic FMH, shows generalized villous edema, with

Fig. 13. Histopathology of complete hydatidiform mole. (*A*) Chorionic villi are avascular, and demonstrate large cisterns and abundant trophoblastic proliferation (original magnification ×40). (*B*) Higher magnification reveals extensive trophoblastic proliferation and patchy cellular atypia and (*C*) that the proliferation includes both cytotrophoblasts and syncytiotrophoblast (original magnification ×100). (*From* Heller DS. Gestational trophoblastic disease. In: McManus LW, Mitchell RN, editors. Pathobiology of human disease: a dynamic encyclopedia of disease mechanisms. Philadelphia: Elsevier; in press.)

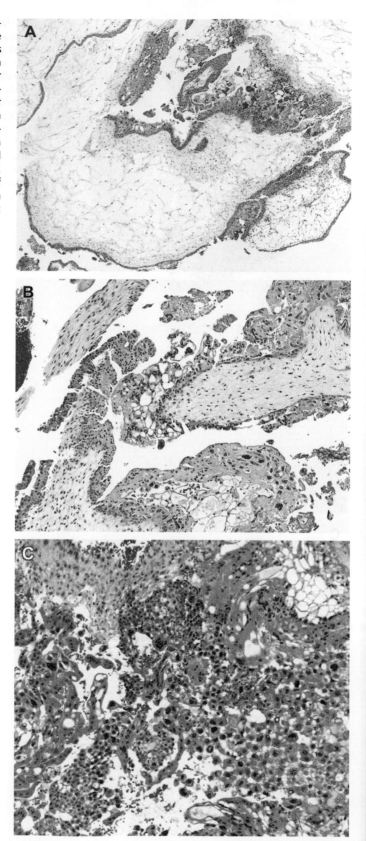

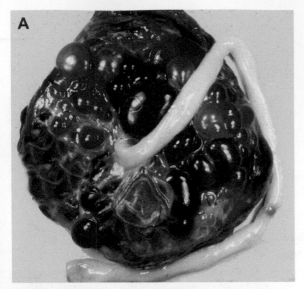

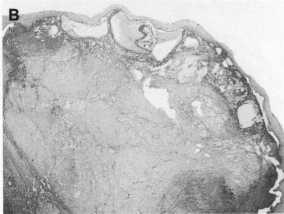

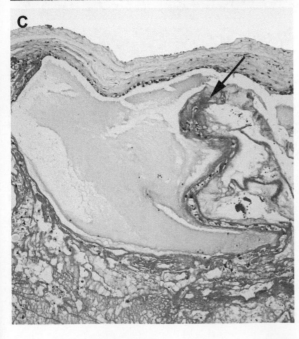

Fig. 14. Subchorionic cysts/thrombohematomas. (*A*) Gross image of multiple, bulging subchorionic cysts containing serous to proteinaceous fluid. Some contain degenerating, maternal blood products and are discolored brown-green. (*B*) Microscopically, the cysts are lined by cytotrophoblasts and often have thrombohematomas at their base (original magnification ×40). (*C*) Higher magnification further demonstrates breakdown of a cyst wall (*arrow*) with leakage of blood into the cyst space (original magnification ×100). ([A] *From* Baergen RN. Manual of pathology of the human placenta. 2nd edition. New York: Springer; 2011. p. 222, Fig. 14.5; with permission.)

orthochromic normoblastemia (circulating excessive numbers of NRBCs, with small, perfectly round, "ink dot" nuclei in a rim of brightly eosinophilic cytoplasm) or frank erythroblastosis (circulating, fetal NRBC precursors with a larger nucleocytoplasmic ratio, and more basophilic cytoplasm) (see **Fig. 11A, B**). Immature intermediate and distal villi are affected, but mature stem and intermediate villi are relatively spared, because of their collagenous stroma. Cistern formation and the ectatic anomalous vessels of PMD are absent. FMH is detected clinically, by Kleihauer-Betke or flow cytometric methodologies, but histologic examination may reveal numerous NRBCs in the perivillous space, and their fetal origin can be confirmed by immunohistochemical stains for fetal hemoglobin (see **Fig. 11C**).

DIAGNOSIS OF PMD

The diagnosis of PMD should be made when the placenta is large for gestational dates and has cirsoid, tortuous, variably thrombosed, and poorly ramifying vessels on the chorionic plate; an excessively long and/or coiled umbilical cord; myxomatous, thickened stem villi with redundant, ropey, ectatic vessels; and hydropic-appearing villi scattered amidst more normal-appearing, chorionic villous tissue. PMD should also be considered when gross or microscopic findings suggest a partial hydatidiform mole, but the DNA content is diploid. When obtained, an accompanying clinical history of a nondysmorphic fetus with IUGR or suspected BWS, hepatic mesenchymal hamartoma, or the occurrence of an autosomal recessive disorder for which the father is the only heterozygous carrier is also highly supportive. The main histolopathologic findings of PMD include the following:

1. Chorionic plate and stem villous vascular dilatation and foci of vascular mural attenuation, myxomatous change, with or without luminal compromise attributable to thrombi of varying age
2. Clusters of abnormally vascularized stem villi (light microscopic correlates of grossly seen vascular redundancies)
3. Large to distal branch stem villous stromal hypocellularity and cistern formation
4. Hypervascularized, distal stem, and intermediate villi with concentration of abnormal, thickly muscularized to thrombosed vessels subjacent to the trophoblast (vs the centralized location of vessels seen in normal villi)
5. Hydropic and degenerated villi scattered among intervening more normal-appearing villi

The histopathology of PMD also includes the findings of proximal and more distal stem villous stromal hypercellularity or a more fibromatous appearance, because, although predominantly vascular in expression, the mesenchymal dysplasia of PMD is not limited to vascular proliferative abnormalities and can include marked edema[17] and even the abnormal presence of villous stromal lymphatic differentiation.[31] Foci of distal villous karyorrhexis, erythrocyte extravasation, and sclerosis (distal villous FTVs); perivascular hematoma formation; fetal normoblastemia/erythroblastosis; and features of chorangiosis, chorangioma, and diffuse multifocal chorangiomatosis, are not uncommon.[1,2,4–16] FTVs result in compromise of chorionic villous blood flow and distal villous atrophy. Vascular undulations and attenuations likely explain the occurrence of thrombi and perivascular hematomas and lead to leakage of fetal blood into the chorionic plate, villous stroma, or perivillous space[2,9,19] and/or destruction of fetal erythrocytes. The mural myxomatous areas are likely more permeable and contribute to the accumulations of stromal fluid, but stromal edema is also seen in villi without abnormal vessels. Fetal anemia may be evidenced by normoblastemia to frank erythroblastosis with stress-related dyserythropoiesis, particularly if PMD is complicated by chronic or acute fetomaternal hemorrhage (FMH).[33] FMH may be suspected by the identification of numerous NRBCs in the perivillous space, and immunohistochemical stains for fetal hemoglobin can confirm that the NRBC are of fetal origin (O.M.F.-P. observation). Abnormalities of chorionic villous perfusion and variations in villous blood pressure presumably result in hypoxic stimuli and/or the development of foci of chorangiosis in PMD. The occasional, co-occurrences of chorangioma or sites of chorangiomatosis may reflect a point(s) of overlap in their pathogeneses with PMD, as they likely represent proliferative developmental lesions of immature stem and intermediate villi,[2,3,22,43–46] but, to date, PMD is distinguished by involvement of umbilical cord vessels and chorionic plate and very proximal stem villous vessels.

Androgenetic-biparental mosaicism (ABM), in which a subset of cells in the placenta are diploid but harbor only paternal chromosomes, has been the most consistent molecular alteration observed in PMD.[5,6,16,17,21,24,37–40] The androgenetic cells in ABM have pan-genomic paternal uniparental disomy (paternal alleles and imprinting at all loci), and detection of allelic imbalances consistent with ABM is considered confirmatory evidence for the diagnosis of PMD.[4,7,11,13,17,24,28,41] Studies have revealed that the anomalous, but diploid villi of PMD have androgenetic stromal cells. They have also shown that PMD epithelial trophoblasts are derived from biparental diploid cells bearing the normal complement of maternal and paternal haploid chromosome sets (biparental diploidy).[5,6,16,17,21,24,37–40] In addition to ABM, some cases of PMD may result from a mosaic distribution of placental cells with segmental forms of uniparental disomy, possibly restricted to the BWS locus on chromosome 11p15.5 [24]. Immunohistochemical staining for the *CDKN1C* gene product, p57[KIP2], provides an indirect, light-microscopic assessment for global allelic imbalance in ABM or segmental loss of maternal 11p15.5 imprinting, because the gene p57[KIP2], on chromosome 11p15.5, encodes a cyclin-dependent kinase inhibitor that is expressed from the *maternally* acquired chromosome, but methylated (silenced) on the *paternally* inherited genome.[41] The typical case of PMD shows *absence* of p57[kip2] nuclear immunostaining in portions of the stroma (vascular mural and endothelial cells) of abnormally vascularized stem villi, but *positive* linear staining (presence of the product of the maternally derived active allele) in the overlying villous surface trophoblast. Nondysmorphic villi in the section exhibit nuclear staining within the stroma and trophoblast (normal staining pattern). These findings are consistent with androgenetic allelic imbalance in villi with the morphology of PMD, but not within the normal-appearing villi (**Fig. 15**).

It is important to emphasize that, because the distribution of androgenetic cells and associated PMD histopathology is rarely uniformly present, villous sampling limitations, for molecular genetic or immunohistochemical studies, are a potential issue. On the other hand, if an appropriately sampled case, with convincing PMD histomorphology, but a negative or inconclusive immunohistochemical staining pattern for the p57[KIP2] gene product, is encountered, follow-up molecular genetic studies should be strongly considered. Fluorescence in situ hybridization studies using polymorphic allele-specific probes,[39] provide an alternative approach, but are not as widely practiced as molecular tests that rely on DNA extracts from fresh, frozen, or fixed tissue.[21,53] Notably, the authors have encountered rare cases of histomorphologic PMD, and negative or inconclusive immunohistochemical *and* negative molecular genetic studies. We propose that these atypical cases may represent currently unidentified segmental allelic imbalances, not distinguishable by molecular studies used to evaluate them. Because PMD is associated with high risks for adverse perinatal outcomes and risks of fetal/neonatal hamartomas, we recommend the pathology report include a comment conveying these risks.

Pitfalls
PLACENTAL MESENCHYMAL DYSPLASIA

#1	! Gross appearance of PMD may be confused with a partial hydatidiform mole, as hydropic villi are scattered among normal-appearing villi
	• Presence of ectatic tortuous vessels on chorionic plate with intervening areas of a netlike vascular distribution or more normal-appearing vascular ramification pattern associated with PMD, *not* partial mole
	• Umbilical cord is often excessively long or twisted, with varices in PMD
	• Ropey and myxomatous proximal and distal stem villi typically seen in PMD
	• Diploid karyotype in PMD, triploid in partial mole
#2	! Trophoblast hyperplasia and pseudoinclusions are *not* present in PMD
#3	! Some distal villi may show only edema or cistern formation
#4	! Sampling important for detection of abnormal vasculature and immunohistochemical/molecular alterations of PMD
#5	! Stromal dysplasia not limited to vascular component: increased stromal cellularity and collagen deposition may be present
#6	! Foci of chorangiosis, chorangioma, and chorangiomatosis may be present
	• None of these involves umbilical cord or chorionic plate or primary proximal stem villous vessels

Fig. 15. p57^{kip} immunohistochemistry in PMD. The figure illustrates 2 microscopic fields from a placenta with mesenchymal dysplasia and molecularly proven androgenetic-biparental mosaicism. (A) Swollen edematous villi contain presumed androgenetic stromal cells, which lack p57^{kip}-immunoreactive nuclei; cytoplasmic immunoreactivity in biparental cytotrophoblast cells is retained. (B) A different field shows morphologically normal villi with p57^{kip}-immunoreactive stromal and cytotrophoblast cells, consistent with the mosaic nature of the androgenetic stroma in PMD.

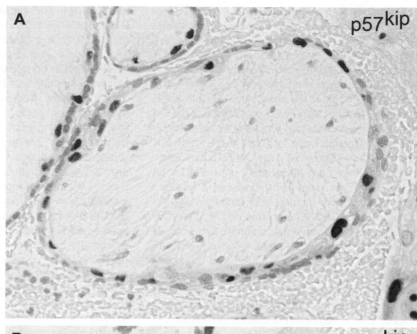

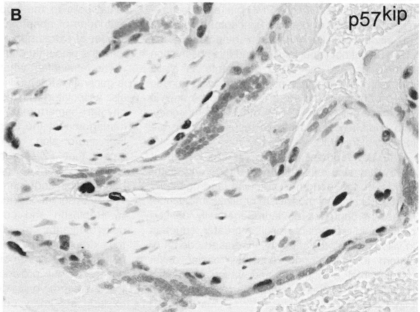

CLINICAL CORRELATIONS AND CLINICOPATHOGENETIC IMPLICATIONS OF PMD

Fetal/neonatal findings and complications with PMD include IUGR, BWS, high risks of morbidity and mortality, visceral hamartomas, and visceral and cutaneous hemangiomas. Despite the presence of placentomegaly, 50% of gestations with PMD are complicated by fetal IUGR. Intrauterine fetal demise (IUFD) occurs in 43% of cases.[3] Excessive cord coiling and/or cord length could also contribute to perturbations in blood flow within the cord or chorionic villous tree, FTVs, or ischemia, and/or result in lethal cord complications, such as obstruction, knots, or prolapse.[2] Increased risks of perinatal morbidity and mortality may also be due to fetomaternal hemorrhage and/or fetal/neonatal coagulopathy.[33]

One-fourth to one-third of cases of PMD are associated with BWS, with fetuses exhibiting composite or select features of the syndrome[17] (macrosomia, hemihyperplasia ["hemihypertrophy"] and visceromegaly, omphalocele, macroglossia, renal anomalies, and adrenal cytomegaly).[3,4,7,11,13,17] The seeming paradox of the association of both IUGR *and* macrosomia, with PMD, probably reflects the specific allelic imbalances involved. As noted previously, the genetic locus for BWS is on 11p15.5,[54] and mosaic segmental loss of 11p15.5 gene imprinting has been associated with PMD,[24] in some instances, presumably because it includes the insulin growth factor-2 (*IGF-2*) (paternally expressed) and *CDKN1C* (encodes p57[kip], paternally silent) genes. Uniparental disomy for paternal 11p15.5, in such cases, could result in cells with unopposed expression of IGF-2 and complete silencing of p57[KIP2]; IGF-2 overexpression and loss of the CDKN1C protein complex, responsible for the arrest of the cell cycle, in G1 phase, would lead to loss of regulation of cellular proliferation in the affected cells. Of note, PMD has also been reported in cases of confined placental mosaicism for trisomy 13 (ie, mosaicism detected in the placenta but not in the fetus),[28] and this observation further suggests that PMD represents an allelic imbalance of imprinting, possibly involving genetic loci on chromosome 13. It remains to be seen if chromosomes 7 or 15, or other chromosomes with imprinted loci, might be responsible, in rare instances, for PMD.

The development of IUGR, in cases without BWS, may also reflect the percentage and distribution of the abnormal villi with androgenetic/biparental stromal mosaicism or allelic imbalance; higher percentages of androgenetically derived cells would presumably result in greater reduction in villous functional capacity, increased edema or cistern formation, and, possibly, earlier onset of placental dysfunction and vascular ectasia. Investigation of the mechanisms by which PMD might arise[5,6,15,17,20,21,23,25,38,39] has yielded strong evidence for two pathways. In one pathway, fertilization is normal, but the subsequent mitoses are abnormal.[17] In the second, a single ovum is fertilized by 2 haploid spermatozoa, with subsequent generation of 2 types of diploid, daughter cells, one of which is normal, and one with paternal disomy.[21] In either scenario, any resulting 46,YY cells would be nonviable, and this likely explains the female preponderance seen in PMD. In addition, the investigations of Robinson and colleagues,[21] indicate that there are many possibilities for the maternal (M1 or M2) and paternal (P1 or P2) make-up of the abnormal cell lines in PMD, depending on the combination of maternal (M) and paternal (P) pronuclei (M1P1/P1P2; M2P1/P1P2; M1P1/P1P1; M1P2/P2P2; M2P1/P1P2, and so forth) that contribute to the androgenetic and biparental lineages, respectively. Specific combinations may result in poorer placental function and IUGR.

In the cases studied, androgenetic/biparental mosaicism or allelic imbalance is confined to the placental mesenchyme, and mesodermal overgrowth is evidenced primarily as vascular proliferation, redundancy, and ectasia; the mosaicism appears to be absent or of such limited distribution in the chorionic villus that it is not identifiable in the trophoblast. However, Kaiser-Rogers and colleagues[17] studied term placentas and could not exclude the possibility that androgenetic cells might have contributed to early undifferentiated cytotophoblastic differentiation, but, because of limited ability to differentiate and persist to term, were undetectable. To date, and for reasons that are unclear, it also appears that, in PMD, there is preferential allocation of the biparental cells to the trophoblastic epithelium, and restriction of abnormal androgenetic cells to the subset of extraembryonic mesoderm destined to form the placental chorion.[17]

The fetus/infant whose placenta exhibits PMD, is generally structurally normal; however, PMD is also associated with the presence of infant mesenchymal hamartomas of the liver,[2,12,23,26,32,35] hamartoma of the lung,[32] and hemangiomas of liver and/or skin.[21,42] Recent studies have indicated that *PMD-associated*[23,26,35] and some *sporadic*[42] hepatic mesenchymal hamartomas both exhibit androgenetic/biparental mosaicism. These observations further confirm those made by Robinson and colleagues,[21] that androgenetic/biparental mosaicism is not limited to the extraembryonic mesenchyme. Although, theoretically, the short umbilical stalk of early embryogenesis might provide a migratory access for the extraembryonic cells, investigators cannot exclude a primary contribution of androgenetic cells to intraembryonic mesoderm in embryos with androgenetic/biparental mosaicism.[21,26,42]

SUMMARY

In summary, in most cases, androgenetic cells appear confined to a subset of villous stromal cells in PMD, and, save one report[40] in which the presence of ABM was found in the trophoblast, do not appear to involve the villous epithelium. Androgenetic cells may also be present in infants with placentas with mesenchymal dysplasia, but have not been detected in white blood cells of the limited number of reported cases in which such studies were performed. These infants, although appearing healthy at birth, may have underappreciated risks for developing tumorous growths later in childhood, and, possibly, even adulthood. To date, there are no long-term follow-up studies of infants with placentas with mesenchymal dysplasia. It is unclear whether these individuals might harbor tissues with allelic imbalance and develop hamartomas or neoplasms in these tissues, later in life, as they grow, go through puberty, and/or become individually exposed to environmental factors that affect their cellular processes of proliferation, differentiation, and repair. In addition, the abnormal cell lines with androgenetic *iso*disomy (ie, P1P1 or P2P2) may have worse outcomes than those with androgenetic *hetero*disomy (P1P2) or some other imbalance of imprinting that is more limited to a single chromosome (ie, chromosome 11).[21] Thus, future investigations of PMD may provide insights into the role of ABM and allelic imbalance in fetoplacental maldevelopment, isolated visceral maldevelopment, and adverse pregnancy outcomes. In addition, molecular genetic studies of PMD may shed light on the pathogenetic mechanisms responsible for the rare cases of complete mole exhibiting biparental origin[55,56] or presence of select maternal chromosomes,[57] partial moles that have loss of select maternal chromosome,[58] and cases of persistent gestational trophoblastic disease with placental and fetal ABM.[20]

REFERENCES

1. Umazume T, Kataoka S, Kamamuta K, et al. Placental mesenchymal dysplasia, a case of intrauterine sudden death of fetus with rupture of cirsoid periumbilical chorionic vessels. Diagn Pathol 2011;6:38.
2. Baergen RN. Manual of pathology of the human placenta. 2nd edition. New York: Springer; 2011. p. 220–420.
3. Pham T, Steele J, Stayboldt C, et al. Placental mesenchymal dysplasia is associated with high rates of intrauterine growth restriction and fetal demise: a report of 11 new cases and a review of the literature. Am J Clin Pathol 2006;126:67–78.
4. Paradinas FJ, Sebire NJ, Fisher RA, et al. Pseudo-partial moles: placental stem vessel hydrops and the association with Beckwith-Wiedemann syndrome and complete moles. Histopathology 2001;39:447–54.
5. Thaker HM. The partly molar pregnancy that is not a partial mole. Pediatr Dev Pathol 2005;8:146–7.
6. Sebire NJ, Fisher RA. Partly molar pregnancies that are not partial moles: additional possibilities and implications. Pediatr Dev Pathol 2005;8:732–3.
7. Lage JM. Placentomegaly with massive hydrops of placental stem villi, diploid DNA content, and fetal omphaloceles—possible association with Beckwith-Wiedemann syndrome. Hum Pathol 1991;22:591–7.
8. Lee G, Chi JG, Cha KS. An unusual venous anomaly of the placenta. Am J Clin Pathol 1991;95:48–51.
9. Moscoso G, Jauniaux E, Hustin J. Placental vascular anomaly with diffuse mesenchymal stem villous hyperplasia. A new clinico-pathological entity? Pathol Res Pract 1991;187:324–8.
10. Sander CM. Angiomatous malformation of placental chorionic stem vessels and pseudo-partial molar placentas: report of five cases. Pediatr Pathol 1993;13:621–33.
11. Jauniaux E, Nicolaides KH, Hustin J. Perinatal features associated with placental mesenchymal dysplasia. Placenta 1997;18:701–6.
12. Kitano Y, Ruchelli E, Weiner S, et al. Hepatic mesenchymal hamartoma associated with mesenchymal stem villous hyperplasia of the placenta. Fetal Diagn Ther 2000;15:134–8.
13. Ohyama M, Kojyo T, Gotoda H, et al. Mesenchymal dysplasia of the placenta. Pathol Int 2000;50:759–64.
14. Lokan J, Chan YF, Agnesta F. Placental mesenchymal dysplasia. Pathology 2002;34:375–8.
15. Matsui H, Iitsuka Y, Yamazawa K, et al. Placental mesenchymal dysplasia initially diagnosed as partial mole. Pathol Int 2003;53:810–3.
16. Gibson BR, Muir-Padilla J, Champeaux A, et al. Mesenchymal dysplasia of the placenta. Placenta 2004;25:671–2.
17. Kaiser-Rogers KA, McFadden DE, Livasy CA, et al. Androgenetic/biparental mosaicism causes placental mesenchymal dysplasia. J Med Genet 2006;43:187–92.
18. Surti U, Hill LM, Dunn J, et al. Twin pregnancy with a chimeric androgenetic and biparental placenta in one twin displaying placental mesenchymal dysplasia phenotype. Prenat Diagn 2005;25:1048–56.
19. Mulch AD, Stallings SP, Salafia CM. Elevated maternal serum alpha-fetoprotein, umbilical vein varix, and mesenchymal dysplasia: are they related? Prenat Diagn 2006;26:659–61.
20. Surti U, Hoffner L, Kolthoff M, et al. Persistent gestational trophoblastic disease after an androgenetic/biparental fetal chimera: a case report and review. Int J Gynecol Pathol 2006;25:366–72.
21. Robinson WP, Lauzon JL, Innes AM, et al. Origin and outcome of pregnancies affected by androgenetic/biparental chimerism. Hum Reprod 2007;22:1114–22.
22. Parveen Z, Tongson-Ignacio JE, Fraser CR, et al. Placental mesenchymal dysplasia. Arch Pathol Lab Med 2007;131:131–7.

23. Francis B, Hallam L, Kecskes Z, et al. Placental mesenchymal dysplasia associated with hepatic mesenchymal hamartoma in the newborn. Pediatr Dev Pathol 2007;10:50–4.

24. Robinson WP, Slee J, Smith N, et al. Placental mesenchymal dysplasia associated with fetal overgrowth and mosaic deletion of the maternal copy of 11p15.5. Am J Med Genet A 2007;143:1752–9.

25. Schuetzle MN, Uphoff TS, Hatten BA, et al. Utility of microsatellite analysis in evaluation of pregnancies with placental mesenchymal dysplasia. Prenat Diagn 2007;27:1238–44.

26. Reed RC, Beischel L, Schoof J, et al. Androgenetic/biparental mosaicism in an infant with hepatic mesenchymal hamartoma and placental mesenchymal dysplasia. Pediatr Dev Pathol 2008;11:377–83.

27. H'Mida D, Gribaa M, Yacoubi T, et al. Placental mesenchymal dysplasia with Beckwith-Wiedemann syndrome fetus in the context of biparental and androgenic cell lines. Placenta 2008;29:454–60.

28. Mungen E, Dundar O, Muhcu M, et al. Placental mesenchymal dysplasia associated with trisomy 13: sonographic findings. J Clin Ultrasound 2008; 36:454–6.

29. Ang DC, Rodriguez Urrego PA, Prasad V. Placental mesenchymal dysplasia: a potential misdiagnosed entity. Arch Gynecol Obstet 2009; 279:937–9.

30. Vaisbuch E, Romero R, Kusanovic JP, et al. Three-dimensional sonography of placental mesenchymal dysplasia and its differential diagnosis. J Ultrasound Med 2009;28:359–68.

31. Heazell AE, Sahasrabudhe N, Grossmith AK, et al. A case of intrauterine growth restriction in association with placental mesenchymal dysplasia with abnormal placental lymphatic development. Placenta 2009;30: 654–7.

32. Tortoledo M, Galindo A, Ibarrola C. Placental mesenchymal dysplasia associated with hepatic and pulmonary hamartoma. Fetal Pediatr Pathol 2010; 29:261–70.

33. Sengers FB, van Lijnschoten G, van der Sluijs-Bens JP, et al. Haematological abnormalities in premature babies due to placental mesenchymal dysplasia. Ned Tijdschr Geneeskd 2010;154:A1040 [in Dutch].

34. Starikov R, Goldman R, Dizon DS, et al. Placental mesenchymal dysplasia presenting as a twin gestation with complete molar pregnancy. Obstet Gynecol 2011;118:445–9.

35. Mack-Detlefsen B, Boemers TM, Groneck P, et al. Multiple hepatic mesenchymal hamartomas in a premature associated with placental mesenchymal dysplasia. J Pediatr Surg 2011;46:e23–5.

36. Woo GW, Rocha FG, Gaspar-Oishi M, et al. Placental mesenchymal dysplasia. Am J Obstet Gynecol 2011;205:e3–5.

37. McConnell TG, Murphy KM, Hafez M, et al. Diagnosis and subclassification of hydatidiform moles using p57 immunohistochemistry and molecular genotyping: validation and prospective analysis in routine and consultation practice settings with development of an algorithmic approach. Am J Surg Pathol 2009;33:805–17.

38. Murphy KM, McConnell TG, Hafez MJ, et al. Molecular genotyping of hydatidiform moles: analytic validation of a multiplex short tandem repeat assay. J Mol Diagn 2009;11:598–605.

39. Chiang S, Fazlollahi L, Nguyen A, et al. Diagnosis of hydatidiform moles by polymorphic deletion probe fluorescence in situ hybridization. J Mol Diagn 2011;13:406–15.

40. Makrydimas G, Sebire NJ, Thornton SE, et al. Complete hydatidiform mole and normal live birth: a novel case of confined placental mosaicism: case report. Hum Reprod 2002;17:2459–63.

41. Matsuoka S, Thompson JS, Edwards MC, et al. Imprinting of the gene encoding a human cyclin-dependent kinase inhibitor, p57KIP2, on chromosome 11p15. Proc Natl Acad Sci U S A 1996;93:3026–30.

42. Lin J, Cole BL, Qin X, et al. Occult androgenetic-biparental mosaicism and sporadic hepatic mesenchymal hamartoma. Pediatr Dev Pathol 2011;14: 360–9.

43. Ogino S, Redline RW. Villous capillary lesions of the placenta: distinctions between chorangioma, chorangiomatosis, and chorangiosis. Hum Pathol 2000; 31:945–54.

44. Amer HZ, Heller DS. Chorangioma and related vascular lesions of the placenta—a review. Fetal Pediatr Pathol 2010;29:199–206.

45. Altshuler G. Chorangiosis. An important placental sign of neonatal morbidity and mortality. Arch Pathol Lab Med 1984;108:71–4.

46. Bagby C, Redline RW. Multifocal chorangiomatosis. Pediatr Dev Pathol 2011;14:38–44.

47. Berkowitz RS, Goldstein DP. Clinical practice. Molar pregnancy. N Engl J Med 2009;360:1639–45.

48. Buza N, Hui P. Gestational trophoblastic disease: histopathological diagnosis in the molecular era. Diagn Histopathol 2010;16:526–37.

49. Sebire NJ. Histopathological diagnosis of hydatidiform mole: contemporary features and clinical implications. Fetal Pediatr Pathol 2010;29:1–16.

50. Ronnett BM, DeScipio C, Murphy KM. Hydatidiform moles: ancillary techniques to refine diagnosis. Int J Gynecol Pathol 2011;30:101–16.

51. Heller DS, Rush D, Baergen RN. Subchorionic hematoma associated with thrombophilia: report of three cases. Pediatr Dev Pathol 2003;6:261–4.

52. Tuuli MG, Norman SM, Odibo AO, et al. Perinatal outcomes in women with subchorionic hematoma: a systematic review and meta-analysis. Obstet Gynecol 2011;117:1205–12.

53. Bourque DK, Penaherrera MS, Yuen RK, et al. The utility of quantitative methylation assays at imprinted genes for the diagnosis of fetal and placental disorders. Clin Genet 2011;79:169–75.

54. Ping AJ, Reeve AE, Law DJ, et al. Genetic linkage of Beckwith-Wiedemann syndrome to 11p15. Am J Hum Genet 1989;44:720–3.

55. Fisher RA, Hodges MD. Genomic imprinting in gestational trophoblastic disease—a review. Placenta 2003;24(Suppl A):S111–8.

56. Fisher RA, Hodges MD, Newlands ES. Familial recurrent hydatidiform mole: a review. J Reprod Med 2004;49:595–601.

57. McConnell TG, Norris-Kirby A, Hagenkord JM, et al. Complete hydatidiform mole with retained maternal chromosomes 6 and 11. Am J Surg Pathol 2009;33: 1409–15.

58. DeScipio C, Haley L, Beierl K, et al. Diandric triploid hydatidiform mole with loss of maternal chromosome 11. Am J Surg Pathol 2011;35:1586–91.

Correlation of Placental Pathology with Perinatal Brain Injury

Raymond W. Redline, MD

KEYWORDS

• Perinatal brain injury • Placental pathology • Neurodisability

ABSTRACT

The purpose of placental pathology is to explain adverse clinical outcomes. One of the most tragic of these outcomes is perinatal brain injury with subsequent neurodisability. Findings in the placenta can play an important role in documenting sentinel events, uncovering clinically silent thromboinflammatory disease processes, revealing developmental alterations in functional reserve, and suggesting alterations in related maternal and fetal physiology. These findings, when integrated with clinical data, provide a plausible explanation for an otherwise unexpected outcome and can be helpful for treating physicians and family members.

OVERVIEW: PERINATAL BRAIN INJURY

Cerebral palsy (CP) and related forms of neurodisability related to perinatal brain injury occur in approximately 2 to 3 of 1000 live births.[1] Although the proportion of cases occurring in very low-birth-weight (VLBW) infants is rising, a majority of cases (50%–60%) continue to involve term and near-term gestations delivering after 34 weeks. Overriding risk factors in the VLBW population include developmental immaturity, underlying fetal growth restriction (FGR), cardiopulmonary instability in early neonatal period, and infections occurring before and after birth. Placental pathology in VLBW infants, although important, plays a circumscribed role by determining causes of FGR and identifying significant fetal inflammatory responses (FIR) to infection. The causes of neurodisability in term and near-term infants are less clear

and placental pathology can play a major role in identifying processes that contribute to central nervous system (CNS) injury.

To properly evaluate these placental processes, it is important to document a thorough gross examination and submit an adequate number of sections, sampling each placental compartment. Synoptic elements of an adequate gross examination are listed in **Box 1**. Particularly important are the trimmed weight of the placenta, the color of the fetal surface, and careful examination of the umbilical cord (UC) for length, extent of coiling, color, and type of insertion. Many placentas are adequately sampled with 3 tissue blocks, but cases of gross abnormalities or a clear clinical history of adverse outcome usually require additional sections. At minimum, 2 cross-sections of UC, 1 membrane roll that includes a piece of the attached marginal placental parenchyma, and 2 full-thickness sections taken within the inner two-thirds of the parenchyma are needed. The chorionic plate is more critical than the basal plate, but both should be sampled. One of the parenchymal sections is ideally taken at the UC insertion site.

Systematic evaluation of a specific set of histologic parameters in every placenta is the key to not missing important diagnoses (**Table 1**). Maternal vascular processes are identified by assessing placental weight, fetoplacental weight ratio, UC diameter, altered maternal arterioles in the membrane roll, developmental abnormalities in the basal plate, and villous changes related to partial or complete obstruction of maternal blood flow in the placental parenchyma. Fetal vascular processes are assessed by evaluating the diameter, muscular wall, and luminal patency of large fetal

Department of Pathology, Case Western Reserve University School of Medicine, University Hospitals Case Medical Center, 11100 Euclid Avenue 5, Cleveland, OH 44106, USA
E-mail address: raymondw.redline@UHhospitals.org

Surgical Pathology 6 (2013) 153–180
http://dx.doi.org/10.1016/j.path.2012.11.005
1875-9181/13/$ – see front matter © 2013 Elsevier Inc. All rights reserved.

> **Box 1**
> **Synoptic elements in the gross description**
>
> Trimmed placental weight
>
> Color of fetal surface and UC
>
> Assessment of fragmentation and completeness of basal plate
>
> Length and site of UC insertion (in centimeters from the placental margin)
>
> Documentation and description of firm, hemorrhagic, and cystic lesions

vessels in the UC, chorionic plate, and major stem villi and by recognizing karyorrhexis or absence of capillaries in the dependent distal villous tree. The diagnosis of inflammatory processes involves assessment of the membranes, subchorionic fibrin, and distal villi. Finally, an increase in circulating nucleated red blood cells (NRBCs) should be excluded in all term or near-term placentas.

Table 1
Checklist for histologic evaluation

UC sections	FIR
	Decreased fetal extracellular fluid (Wharton jelly)
Membrane rolls	Meconium changes
	Chorio(amnio)nitis
	Decidual arteriopathy
Chorionic and large stem villous vessels	Inflammation, thrombosis, necrosis, luminal dilatation
Chorionic plate	Pigment-laden macrophages
	Cellular infiltrates in chorion/subchorionic fibrin
Margin and basal plate	Retroplacental hemorrhages, plasma cells, accreta
Villi, low-power magnification (2×–4×)	Overall maturation (immature/slightly immature/mature)
	Regional variations in architecture
	Localized changes in character
	Foci of agglutination
Villi, higher-power examination (10×–40×)	Definitive diagnosis of villous alterations
	Assessment of circulating fetal NRBCs

SENTINEL EVENTS/TOTAL ASPHYXIA

OVERVIEW

Total asphyxia is an important cause of CNS injury, and severe placental perfusion defects resulting in asphyxia are often referred to as *sentinel events*.[2,3] The obstetric syndrome associated with a sentinel event is called *birth asphyxia* and has a specific definition that includes low cord pH and/or elevated base excess. The corresponding depressed neurologic state in a newborn is known as hypoxic-ischemic or, more properly, neonatal, encephalopathy (NE). Although both clinical and experimental studies suggest that a majority of infants born after total asphyxia either die or recover without sequelae, a minority of survivors develop CP, usually of the spastic quadriplegic type with severe associated developmental disabilities.[4] A considerable amount of attention has been paid over the past 20 years to separating cases of pure birth asphyxia from cases of more complex causation. The current consensus is that approximately 15% of CP in term and near-term infants is due to pure birth asphyxia and that 20% of infants presenting with NE have an isolated preceding sentinel event.[5] The remaining cases are of mixed cause and often associated with significant placental pathology. Another consideration in all cases of suspected sentinel events is to exclude conditions that mimic birth asphyxia, such as birth trauma, Rett syndrome, molybdenum cofactor deficiency, and mitochondrial disease.

The 4 major clinical categories of sentinel events are

1. Premature separation of the placenta from the uterus due to abruptio placenta or uterine rupture
2. Obstruction of fetoplacental blood flow due to UC occlusion
3. Fetal hemorrhage
4. Maternal hypotension

The last category is not usually associated with placental findings and is not discussed further.

ABRUPTIO PLACENTA/UTERINE RUPTURE

Abruptio placenta (acute abruption) is caused by rupture of 1 or more of the maternal spiral arteries that supply the placenta. Risk factors include preeclampsia, vasoactive drugs (cocaine and nicotine), and sheer forces associated with trauma or heavy physical labor. Uterine rupture usually occurs in uteri weakened by a previous cesarean section scar. Both result in large retroplacental hemorrhages that deprive the placenta of its maternal blood supply. Uterine rupture is followed by NE in approximately 32% of cases and abruptio placenta in approximately 11%.[3] Maternal blood in these conditions can escape through the vagina, remain adherent to the uterus, or become embedded in the placenta. It is only in the last situation that a definitive diagnosis of abruptio placenta/uterine rupture can be made by pathologic examination. For these reasons, in cases where a cesarean section is performed, a clinician's observations of uterine rupture or blood clots in the uterine cavity should be considered the gold standard for diagnosis.

Gross findings consistent with abruptio placenta/uterine rupture are adherent, centrally located retroplacental blood clots that either indent or rupture through the basal plate. Occasionally, a compression crater in the basal plate is diagnostic even in the absence of a large clot. The parenchyma overlying a true retroplacental hematoma is often slightly firm. Microscopic features that support the diagnosis include interstitial hemorrhage within the decidua (**Fig. 1**), spread of blood behind the placental membranes, rupture through the basal plate, basal intervillous thrombi/hemorrhages, and alterations in overlying villi, including congestion, edema, and stromal hemorrhage (**Fig. 2**).

COMPLETE UC OCCLUSION

Conditions associated with complete UC occlusion include prolapse, fetal entanglements, overhand knots, and torsion (see the article by Chan elsewhere in this issue). A localized UC lesion (indentation, stricture, or knot) with differing appearance proximal and distal to the site of presumed occlusion is the strongest indicator of compromise (**Fig. 3**). Gross abnormalities placing the UC at risk include excessive length and unprotected vessels at the insertion site (membranous or furcate insertion). In general, the umbilical vein is collapsed before the arteries so a histologic section taken near the UC insertion site may show preferential dilatation of umbilical, chorionic plate, and major stem villous veins relative to arteries (**Fig. 4**). A ratio of greater than 4:1 for venous compared with arterial diameter is proposed for diagnosis.[6] Many of these findings are nonspecific and need to interpreted in the context of clinical data, such as a history of birth asphyxia or a UC blood gas pattern suggestive of obstructed venous blood flow (higher pH and lower base excess in venous compared with arterial blood).[7]

FETAL HEMORRHAGE

Significant fetal hemorrhage can be separated into 2 groups: fetomaternal hemorrhage (FMH) and lacerations involving large fetal vessels. FMH is the more common and occurs due to rupture of distal villi with fetal capillary bleeding into the maternal circulation. Up to 75% of pregnancies are estimated to have FMH of less than 1 mL.[8] The prevalence of massive FMH is probably approximately 1 to 3 of 1000, as determined by

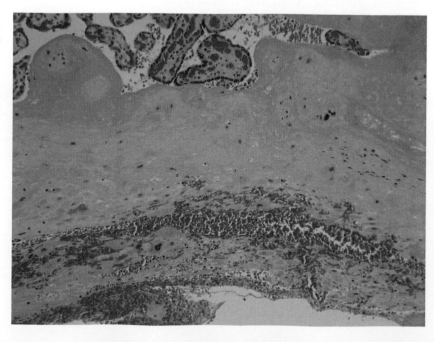

Fig. 1. Acute abruption, decidual interstitial hemorrhage. Dissection of blood between decidual stromal cells in the basal plate is one of the substantiating features that support a diagnosis of abruptio placenta (H&E stain, original magnification 10×).

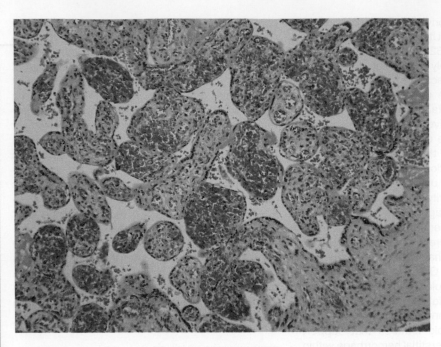

Fig. 2. Acute abruption, villous stromal hemorrhage. Acute ischemic injury can disrupt villous capillaries resulting in fresh stromal hemorrhage (H&E stain, original magnification 10×).

routine testing in Rh-negative pregnancies for determining the need for postpartum Rho(D) immune globulin administration. Massive FMH may present as either stillbirth or a sentinel event. It is estimated that 14% of unexplained stillbirths have significant FMH and a Kleihauer-Betke test or flow cytometric estimation of maternal circulating fetal hemoglobin containing cells is recommended

for all pregnancies with unexpected adverse outcomes.

Lacerations of large fetal vessels are less common and usually involve unprotected vessels that are torn at the time of membrane rupture (ruptured vasa previa). Pregnancies at risk include those with membranous insertion of UC, accessory lobes with bridging vessels, or aberrant membranous vessels

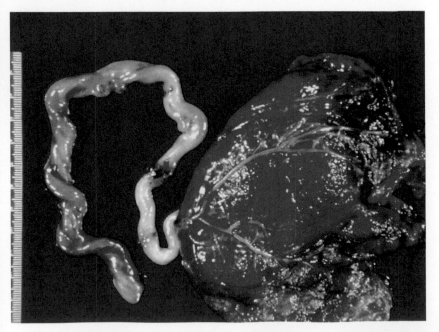

Fig. 3. UC prolapse. Compression of the UC sufficient to occlude fetal vascular blood flow, in this case by trapping between the descending fetal head and the maternal pelvic brim, often results in an abrupt change in color and diameter, as seen at the left.

Fig. 4. UC occlusion. Discordant dilatation of chorionic veins (vein is identified by location below the artery). This pattern develops due to collapse of the umbilical vein and retained flow in the umbilical arteries (H&E stain, original magnification 4×).

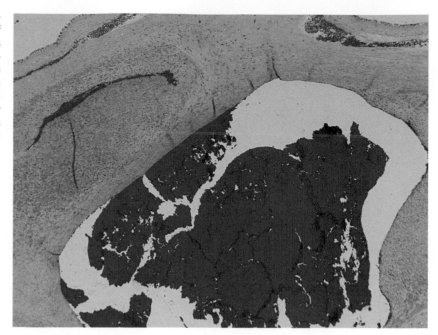

associated with peripheral UC insertion. Other rare causes of laceration are excessive tension on the UC during fetal descent, meconium-induced UC ulceration, and iatrogenic injuries to large vessels during diagnostic procedures.

Intervillous thrombi/hemorrhages (spherical hemorrhages in varying stages of organization completely surrounded by villi) have been shown to represent sites of FMH (**Fig. 5**).[9] Although usually sealed off by coagulated maternal blood, the finding of multiple and/or large intervillous thrombi/hemorrhages increases the risk of significant FMH.[10] The finding of markedly increased circulating fetal NRBCs, suggesting preceding episodes of hemorrhage, can be helpful. A characteristic finding with acute fetal hypovolemia is extreme arteriolar constriction and venular dilation within stem and intermediate villi (**Fig. 6**).

Fig. 5. Intervillous thrombus/hemorrhage. These parenchymal hemorrhagic lesions are surrounded by villi without intervening decidua or trophoblast. The terms, thrombi and hemorrhage, are misnomers. They are extravascular and hence not true thrombi, and, although originating as small FMH, they are predominantly composed of clotted maternal blood that acts to prevent fetal hemorrhage (H&E stain, original magnification 2×).

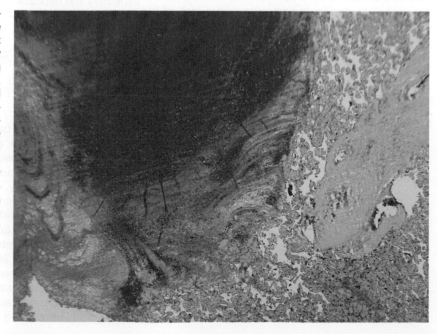

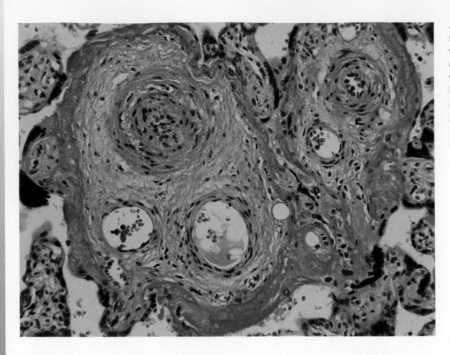

Fig. 6. Stem villous arteriolar constriction and venular dilatation. These changes are often seen with profound fetal blood loss (H&E stain, original magnification 20×).

PITFALLS/DIFFERENTIAL DIAGNOSIS

The differential diagnosis of abruptio placenta/uterine rupture includes recent marginal abruption, hemorrhages occurring after delivery, and artifactual adherence of blood accompanying the placenta in the specimen container (**Box 2**). Acute marginal abruptions are usually small and have their epicenter at the placental margin. Postpartum hemorrhages are sometimes associated with torn or incomplete placentas. The best criteria for excluding significant hemorrhage, are lack of evidence suggesting forceful spread and absence of associated changes in the overlying villi. The differential diagnosis of UC occlusion includes localized UC abnormalities, such as false knots (venous varicosities), focal myxoid degeneration of Wharton jelly, and localized redundancy (switchbacks) of cord vessels leading to nodular thickening of the UC. The differential diagnosis of clinically significant fetal vessel laceration is artifactual tearing after delivery. Lack of adjacent hemorrhage and correlation with clinical history, especially the neonatal hematocrit, are important in this distinction.

Box 2
Sentinel events
Key Features
Extension/spread of hemorrhage
Large or atypically located intervillous thrombi/hemorrhages
Abrupt changes in parenchymal color and texture
Preferential dilatation of chorionic veins
Abrupt changes in UC diameter and color
Pitfalls/Differential Diagnosis
Failure to correlate with clinical history
Changes occurring after delivery of fetus
Torn or fragmented placenta
Localized marginal retroplacental blood clots

PLACENTAL SYNDROMES: FETAL VASCULOPATHIES

OVERVIEW

Many studies over the past 20 years have highlighted the significance and high prevalence of thromboinflammatory lesions involving large fetoplacental vessels in adverse fetal outcomes, including neurodisability.[11–13] In addition to obliterating functional placental parenchyma, these processes lead to the release of cytokines, alarmins, activated coagulation components, and complement into the fetal circulation. The profound and long-lasting effects of such systemic activators has been termed, *genomic storm.*[14] Redistribution of fetoplacental blood flow and fetal thromboembolism may also contribute to adverse outcomes in some cases.

FETAL THROMBOTIC VASCULOPATHY

Definition/Pathogenesis

Fetal thrombotic vasculopathy FTV is defined by degenerative changes in villi downstream to occlusive thrombi in chorionic or major stem villous vessels.[11] Risk factors include the Virchow triad of vessel wall damage, hypercoagulability, and vascular stasis. Thrombi developing due to vessel damage are not considered part of the FTV spectrum and are discussed below. Hypercoagulable states, including antiphospholipid antibody syndrome, maternal diabetes, and thrombophilic mutations, play an etiologic role in some cases of FTV, but most studies suggest that stasis due to UC obstruction or fetal cardiovascular insufficiency is the most common underlying risk factor.[15,16]

Relation to CNS Injury

FTV is associated with NE, CP, and developmental delay in term infants and neuronal injury in stillborns.[12,13,17] One study suggests that infants with NE whose placentas have FTV respond less well to head cooling.[18] A few studies have also implicated FTV in preterm CNS injury and perinatal stroke.[19–21]

Pathologic Characteristics

By gross examination, engorged or discolored chorionic surface vessels containing thrombi or pale firm areas of villous parenchyma

corresponding to regions of avascular villi may be observed in some cases. Even after histologic examination, however, thrombi are documented in only 10% to 30% of FTV. Diagnosis, therefore, depends on recognition of the downstream sequela of thrombotic occlusion; degenerative changes in distal villi (**Figs. 7** and **8**), and involutional changes in intervening intermediate-sized vessels (**Fig. 9**). Degenerative villous changes include hyalinization and absence of capillaries (avascular villi) and necrosis of endothelial, stromal, and red blood cells (stromal vascular karyorrhexis or hemorrhagic endovasculitis). Involutional changes include fibromuscular sclerosis of arteries and fibrous luminal obliteration of veins. A numeric threshold for the diagnosis of FTV has been proposed: 1 or more foci of 10 or more contiguous affected villi plus an overall average of at least 15 affected villi per parenchymal section.[22]

CHRONIC VILLITIS WITH OBLITERATIVE FETAL VASCULOPATHY

Definition/Pathogenesis

Chronic villitis (also known as villitis of unknown etiology [VUE]) is a maternal type 1 delayed-type hypersensitivity allograft reaction to fetal antigens in the distal villous tree observed in approximately 5% to 10% of term placentas (see the article by Faye-Petersen and Kapur elsewhere in this issue).[23] VUE sometimes spreads to involve

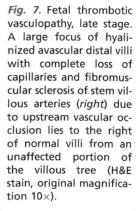

Fig. 7. Fetal thrombotic vasculopathy, late stage. A large focus of hyalinized avascular distal villi with complete loss of capillaries and fibromuscular sclerosis of stem villous arteries (*right*) due to upstream vascular occlusion lies to the right of normal villi from an unaffected portion of the villous tree (H&E stain, original magnification 10×).

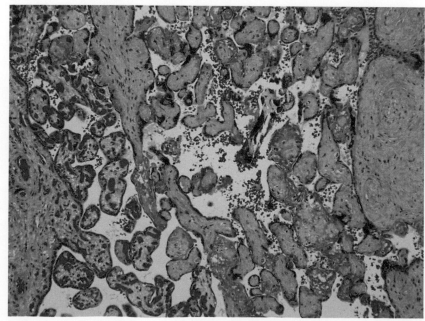

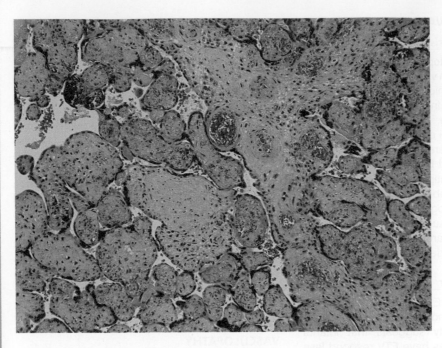

Fig. 8. Fetal thrombotic vasculopathy, early stage. Distal villi show degenerating capillaries, stromal vascular karyorrhexis, and a nonspecific mononuclear cell infiltrate. Larger fetal vessels at the right show fibromuscular sclerosis and luminal fibrosis (H&E stain, original magnification 10×).

proximal villi or even the chorionic plate. When the muscular walls of large fetal vessels become involved, vascular occlusion and downstream villous degeneration constitute a lesion called obliterative fetal vasculopathy (OFV).

Relation to CNS Injury

VUE/OFV is a strong risk factor for CP and NE.[13,20] High-grade VUE alone (see below) also is associated with a variety of other forms of CNS injury, including neonatal seizures and perinatal stroke.[21,24]

Pathologic Characteristics

Placentas with VUE are often small for gestational age and may show patchy ill-defined areas of parenchymal firmness due to perivillous fibrin (PVF) or villous stromal fibrosis. Microscopically,

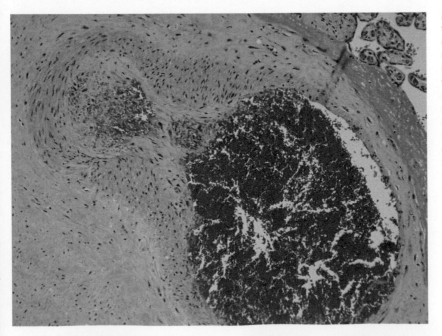

Fig. 9. Large stem villous vein with dilatation and evolving luminal fibrous obliteration; changes seen between the site of thrombotic obstruction and distal avascular villi (H&E stain, original magnification 10×).

Fig. 10. High grade chronic villitis (VUE). Active chronic inflammation involves more than 10 contiguous villi in the upper portion of the figure. Avascular villi, some surrounded by inflammatory fibrin, in the lower portion are suggestive of OFV (H&E stain, original magnification 4×) (see **Fig. 11**).

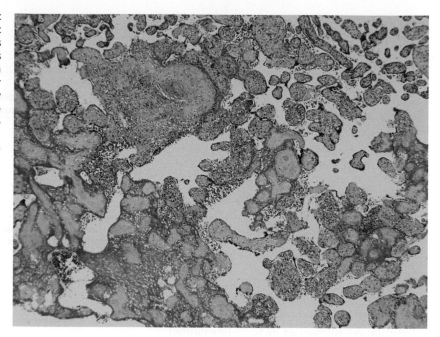

VUE is defined by the presence of T lymphocytes within the villous stroma. The identification of pale, blue-staining aggregates of villi, often with accompanying PVF, at scanning magnification is key for recognizing VUE. A significant component of intervillous inflammation surrounding affected villi may be seen and may include an active neutrophilic or granulomatous component. In most cases, VUE is either low grade (fewer than 10 villi per focus) or exclusively basal in distribution.[23] High-grade VUE (more than 10 contiguous nonbasal villi) is associated with a higher risk of FGR and is more likely to develop OFV (**Fig. 10**). VUE/OFV is characterized by lymphocytic infiltration of stem villi, perivascular adventitial fibrosis, luminal compromise, and degenerative villous changes similar to those seen with FTV (**Fig. 11**).

Fig. 11. VUE with OFV. This stem villus shows severe perivasculitis with concentric fibrosis, active chronic inflammation, luminal narrowing, and early thrombosis. Distal villi would be expected to show degenerative stromal-vascular changes (H&E stain, original magnification 20×).

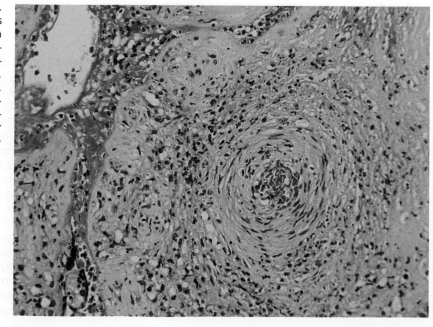

> **Box 3**
> **Fetal vasculopathies**
>
> Key Features
>
> | | Large-Vessel Thrombi | Large-Vessel Inflammatory Cells | Large-Vessel Necrosis | Chorionic Plate Inflammation | Villous Inflammation | Villous Degeneration |
> |---|---|---|---|---|---|---|
> | FTV | ++ | — | — | — | — | ++ |
> | VUE/OFV | Rare | T cells, mΦ | — | Rare | ++ | ++ |
> | ACA (Gr 2 FIR) | Rare | Neutrophils | + | Neutrophils | — | — |
> | MAVN | — | Pigmented mΦ | ++ | Pigmented mΦ | — | — |
> | Eos/T Vasculitis | Rare | T cells, eos | — | — | — | Rare |
>
> *Abbreviations:* ACA, acute chorioamnionitis; Eos, eosinophilic; FTV, fetal thrombotic vasculopathy; Gr 2 FIR, grade 2 fetal inflammatory response; mΦ, macrophage; MAVN, meconium-associated vascular necrosis; T vasculitis, T-cell vasculitis; VUE/OFV, chronic villitis with obliterative vasculopathy.
>
> Pitfalls/Differential Diagnosis
>
> Coexisting FTV and focal VUE without OFV
>
> Villous degenerative changes in stillborns
>
> Avascular villi surrounded by fibrin (involution)

PITFALLS/DIFFERENTIAL DIAGNOSIS

FTV and VUE/OFV can be confused with one another when the predominant feature is extensive avascular villi (**Box 3**). Features favoring FTV include minimal VUE and thrombi in otherwise normal vessels. Features favoring OFV are high-grade VUE and lymphocytes in the proximal villi. Other associated features, such as decidual plasma cells or PVF, also suggest VUE. In difficult cases, a CD3 immunostain may highlight subtle T-cell infiltration. Diffuse involutional changes after stillbirth make diagnosis of FTV or VUE/OFV difficult. Lymphocytic infiltrates indicate underlying VUE whereas areas of villi with degenerative changes more advanced than expected for the estimated duration of fetal death suggest underlying FTV. Finally, other types of fetal vascular inflammation mimic OFV. FIR in chorioamnionitis (discussed later) is limited to the chorionic plate, exclusively neutrophilic and not associated with downstream villous degeneration. Eosinophilic/T-cell vasculitis, a rare idiopathic lesion characterized by infiltration of stem villous and chorionic vessel walls by eosinophils and T lymphocytes, is occasionally associated with thrombosis and downstream villous degeneration (**Fig. 12**).[25] There is generally no villous inflammation, however, and eosinophils are not seen in isolated VUE/OFV.

PLACENTAL SYNDROMES: PROLONGED PARTIAL ASPHYXIA/CHRONIC INTERMITTENT HYPOXIA

OVERVIEW

A second major pattern of brain injury, described by Myers,[2] is prolonged partial asphyxia, elicited experimentally in primates by the application of repetitive, hypoxic events via partial constriction of the maternal aorta. These maneuvers resulted in more survivors, but an increased proportion had significant CNS damage often affecting the basal ganglia. Similar outcomes were observed in sheep after repetitive UC compression.[26] Although difficult to evaluate in human pregnancies, Clapp and coworkers[27] documented neurodevelopmental abnormalities at 1 year of age in infants with UC entanglements in more than 1 antenatal ultrasound. Episodes of FMH also sometimes occur intermittently over a prolonged time period. Whether injury in these situations is the consequence of the additive effects of multiple small insults or due to preconditioning where an

Fig. 12. Eosinophilic/T-cell vasculitis. Large fetal vessel with an intense inflammatory infiltrate centered in the subintimal connective tissue. The mixture of eosinophils and T cells is unique to this lesion (H&E stain, original magnification 40×).

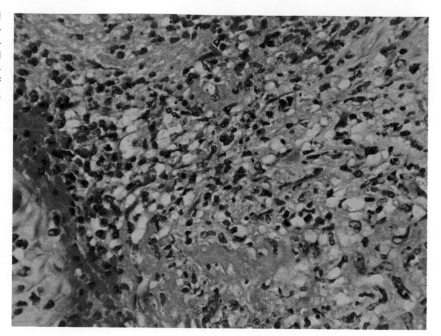

initial insult sensitizes the CNS for an enhanced response after a second hit is not known.

FINDINGS CONSISTENT WITH CHRONIC PARTIAL/INTERMITTENT UC COMPRESSION

Definition/Pathogenesis

Umbilical blood vessels are protected from compression by Wharton jelly, a noncompressible hydrated gel lying between the vessel walls and the epithelial surface. Three conditions predispose to chronic partial/intermittent UC compression:

1. Abnormal insertion: membranous, furcate, or tethered by an amnionic web
2. Changes in architecture: decreased Wharton jelly or hypercoiling
3. Entanglements: fetal nuchal or body coils or UC knots

Because the umbilical vein is more easily collapsed than the arteries, subtotal compression leads to placental congestion and impaired delivery of oxygenated blood to the fetus.

Relation to CNS Injury

Pathologic findings suggestive of chronic UC compression are associated with neuronal damage in stillborn fetuses and both CP and NE in liveborn infants.[18,28,29] Although highly prevalent in infants with neurodisability, ranging from 34% to 43% in various studies, these pathologic changes are less specific than those observed with the fetal vasculopathies and less well supported by clinical history than those found with sentinel events.

Pathologic Characteristics

Gross findings increasing the risk of vascular compression are UC diameter less than 8 mm, 5 or more horizontal UC coils per 10-cm segment, and long UC (more than 70 cm). Histologic findings supporting physiologically significant obstruction include preferential dilatation of large fetal veins compared with adjacent arteries (see **Fig. 4**), intimal fibrin cushions composed of pressure-related deposition of fibrin or fibrinoid material in the intima of large fetal veins (**Fig. 13**), and, most typically, small clusters (less than 10) of avascular villi developing due to reduced flow to the most distal portions of the villous tree (**Fig. 14**).

SUBACUTE AND/OR CHRONIC ABRUPTION

Definition/Pathogenesis

The term, *abruption*, is used to describe at least 4 distinct events.[30–32] The first, acute abruption or abruptio placenta, was discussed previously. The second, acute marginal abruption, is an important cause of preterm delivery but, because of its localized nature and immediate progression to delivery, is rarely associated with CNS injury. The other two, subacute abruption and chronic marginal abruption, both cause intermittent hypoxia.

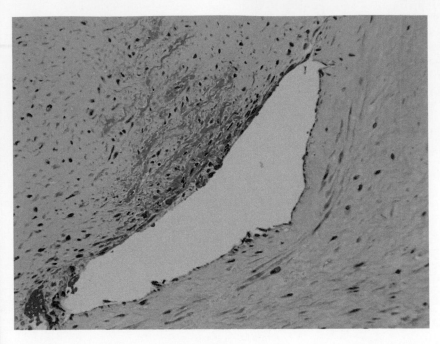

Fig. 13. Recent intimal fibrin cushion. Eccentric aggregate of laminated, eosinophilic fibrin, or fibrinoid within the wall of a large fetal vein exposed to increased intramural pressure (H&E stain, original magnification 20×).

Relation to CNS Injury

Subacute abruption is related to CNS injury in stillborns. Although few doubt its contribution to CNS damage in liveborns, there are no studies that have systematically investigated this relationship. Chronic abruption, alternatively, defined clinically by vaginal bleeding before the third trimester or

pathologically by the finding of chorioamnionic hemosiderosis, was an independent risk factor for CP at term in 2 studies.[33,34]

Pathologic Characteristics

Subacute abruption, like acute abruptio placenta, is an arterial lesion usually occurring in the central

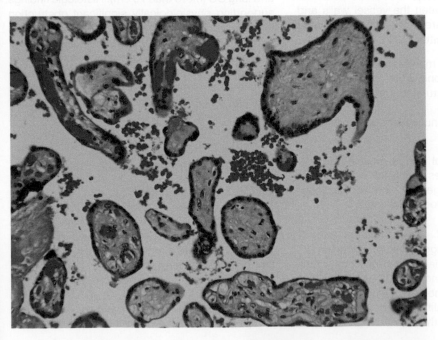

Fig. 14. Small foci of avascular villi suggestive of obstructed UC blood flow. Widely scattered small groups of villi at the most distal portions of the villous tree show advanced degenerative changes (H&E stain, original magnification 4×).

portion of the basal plate. It is characterized by localized central retroplacental hemorrhage with indentation of the basal plate and overlying recent villous infarction (collapse of the intervillous space, villous agglutination, eosinophilia of villous trophoblast, and accumulation of karyorhectic debris in the intervillous space [**Fig. 15**]). Chronic abruption (also known as chronic peripheral separation) is a venous lesion leading to hemorrhage that accumulates at the placental margin or extends medially under the chorionic plate. It is associated with organizing marginal hematomas, circumvallate membrane insertions, and an ultrasound diagnosis of subchorionic hematoma. Microscopically, hemosiderin is often observed near the hematoma and if bleeding extends through the amnion, hemosiderin deposition may extend throughout the placental membranes (diffuse chorioamnionic hemosiderosis) (**Fig. 16**).

PITFALLS/DIFFERENTIAL DIAGNOSIS

The differential diagnosis of chronic/partial intermittent UC obstruction includes artifactual dilatation of large veins and placental congestion due to early UC cord clamping, especially after cesarean sections. Other findings, such as intimal fibrin cushions and small foci of avascular villi, are sometimes seen in FTV, which, as discussed previously, is often related to stasis caused by UC compression. In FTV, more typical thrombi and/or larger foci of degenerating villi are also seen. A

diagnosis of chronic/partial intermittent UC obstruction is strengthened by additional supportive evidence, such as a history of cord entanglement, a UC blood gas pattern consistent with obstructed venous blood flow, or increased circulating fetal NRBCs (discussed later), is helpful.

Spiral artery thrombi also cause recent infarction, but there should not be any retroplacental hemorrhage. Circumvallation is a developmental variation, but in this situation there should be no organizing clot or hemosiderin. Other types of pigment, such as meconium or lipofuschin, mimic hemosiderin. A positive iron stain confirms hemosiderosis, but a negative stain does not exclude chronic abruption since up to 30% of otherwise typical hemosiderin crystals are Prussian blue negative.[35]

PLACENTAL SYNDROMES: UTEROPLACENTAL INSUFFICIENCY/DECREASED PLACENTAL RESERVE

OVERVIEW

It is estimated that the placenta possesses approximately 30% and 40% more capacity for gas exchange than is used in the course of most pregnancies.[10] For this reason, complications of uteroplacental insufficiency are usually limited to impaired fetal growth. Decreased placental reserve, however, can become critical if additional significant stresses are experienced later in

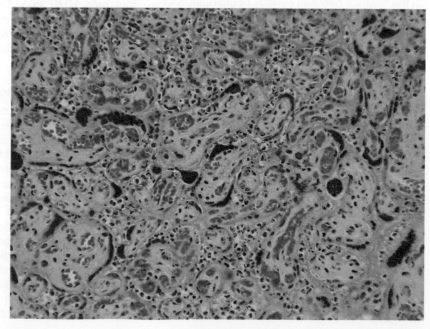

Fig. 15. Subacute abruption, recent villous infarct. Villous parenchyma shows ischemic necrosis with focal loss of trophoblast basophilia, collapse of the intervillous space, and accumulation of necrotic cell fragments and neutrophils. Villous stroma is relatively preserved (H&E stain, original magnification 10×).

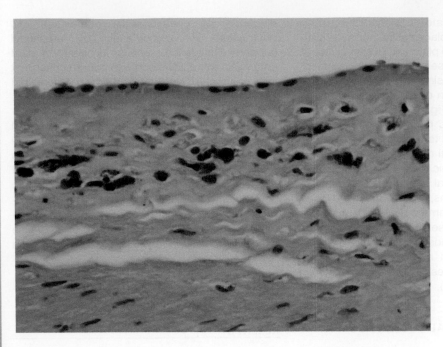

Fig. 16. Chronic abruption, diffuse chorioamnionic hemosiderosis. Marginal hemorrhages can disrupt the integrity of the amnion leading to blood in the amniotic fluid and hemosiderin deposition in the amnion and superficial chorion (H&E stain, original magnification 40×).

gestation. These stressors may be other placental lesions or extraplacental processes, such as maternal hypotension, metabolic stress (diabetes or hypothyroidism), transient hypoxia (uterine hyperstimulation), or hyperthermia (extraplacental infections and epidural anesthesia). Severe variants of lesions in this category can also directly cause neurodisability independent of later stressors. Correlation with CNS injury depends on the balance between severity of uteroplacental insufficiency and the magnitude, timing, and number of the subsequent perinatal stressors.

MATERNAL MALPERFUSION (ACCELERATED MATURATION)

Definition/Pathogenesis

Pathologic changes consistent with maternal malperfusion (MMP) reflect abnormal intervillous blood flow due to inadequate remodeling of the uterine spiral arteries.[36] This defect is part of a more generalized failure in extravillous trophoblast maturation that results in superficial placental implantation and impaired fetal growth and development.[37] Complete obstruction leads to villous infarcts and, in some cases, rupture of the obstructed artery and abruptio placenta. Partially obstructed spiral artery flow results in a stereotypical pattern of changes in distal villous architecture and morphology. In preterm placentas, some of these features recapitulate

findings seen at term, leading to use of the descriptive term, *accelerated maturation*.

Relation to CNS Injury

Villous infarcts are related to CNS injury in stillborns.[38] In a large well-designed epidemiologic study, limited only by exclusively gross pathologic examination, infarcts were a significant risk factor for CP after NE at term.[39] Some evidence suggests that mild MMP in VLBW infants may actually exert a protective effect against CNS injury, whereas more severe forms are risk factors for CP, NE, developmental delay, and abnormal head ultrasound.[40,41]

Pathologic Characteristics

Placentas with MMP are commonly small for gestational age and exhibit an increased fetoplacental weight ratio. The UC is often thin and sometimes peripherally inserted and firm lesions are seen corresponding to villous infarcts. Villous infarcts are histologically characterized by collapse of the intervillous space, ischemic necrosis of villous trophoblast, atrophy of villous stromal vascular elements, and karyorrhectic debris (**Fig. 17**). With MMP, the placental parenchyma at scanning magnification shows a distinctive exaggeration of the normal lobular architecture characterized by alternating areas of villous undergrowth (distal villous hypoplasia) and villous crowding (focal agglutination, increased syncytial knots, and

Fig. 17. Remote villous infarct. Villous parenchyma shows collapse and replacement of the intervillous space by fibrin. Villi show stromal fibrosis and decreased trophoblast basophilia. Fetal capillaries are involuted, but, unlike fetal thrombotic vasculopathy, larger fetal vessels and villous stromal cells persist (H&E stain, original magnification 10×).

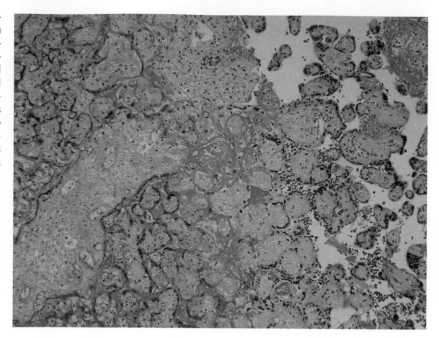

adherent intervillous fibrin not completely surrounding individual villi) (**Figs. 18** and **19**). Other features common in placentas with MMP include decidual arteriopathy (mural hypertrophy or acute atherosis), laminar membrane necrosis, and features of deficient extravillous trophoblast maturation (persistent muscularization of basal plate arteries, basal plate trophoblast giant cells, and chorionic cysts in the membranes, chorionic plate, or parenchyma).

Fig. 18. Changes consistent with MMP (scanning magnification). Partial obstruction of maternal arterial blood flow leads to a typical alternating pattern of distal villous hypoplasia/undergrowth (*right*) and focal villous crowding with villous agglutination, increased syncytial knots, and intervillous fibrin (*left*) (H&E stain, original magnification 4×).

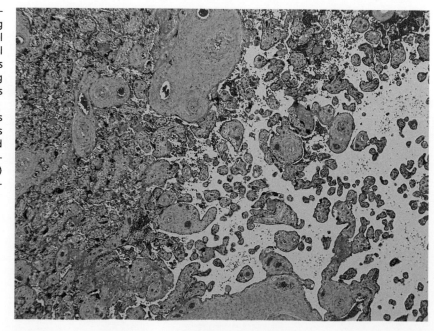

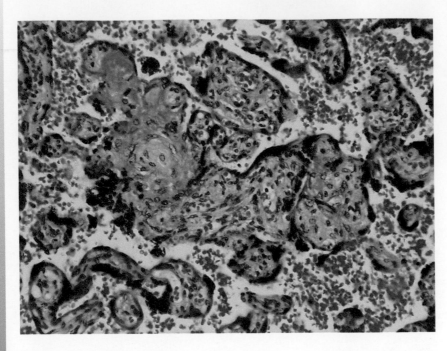

Fig. 19. Changes consistent with MMP (high magnification). Distal villi show decreased diameter, stromal fibrosis, large irregular syncytial knots, and agglutination with significant regions of denuded trophoblast and adherent fibrin (H&E stain, original magnification 20×).

DISTAL VILLOUS IMMATURITY (DELAYED VILLOUS MATURATION)

Definition/Pathogenesis

Distal villous immaturity (DVI), also known as placental maturation defect, is defined as a retarded pattern of villous development.[42] In some ways it is considered the converse of accelerated maturation. It is characterized by excessive villous stroma, deficiencies in the normal intimate relationship of villous capillaries to syncytiotrophoblast (vasculosyncytial membranes), a thickened cellular layer of syncytiotrophoblast, and persistent, occasionally proliferative, cytotrophoblast (**Figs. 20** and **21**). All of these features increase the diffusion distance for oxygen and

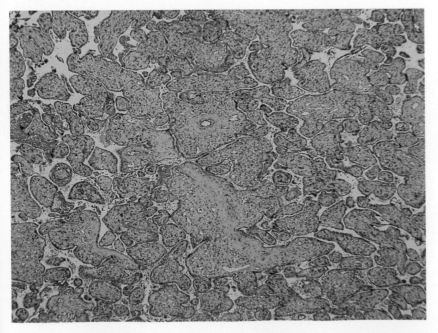

Fig. 20. DVI with patchy multifocal chorangiomatosis. (H&E stain, original magnification 4×) Distal villi show increased diameter, abundant stroma, and many central capillaries. (Hypercapillarization around muscularized fetal vessels in intermediate and stem villi defines chorangiomatosis.)

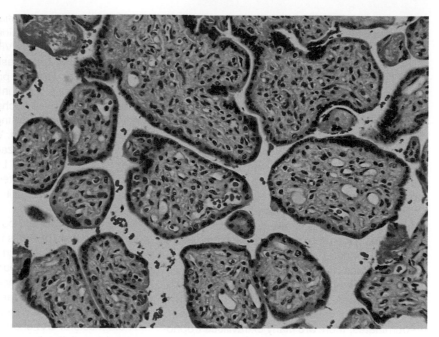

Fig. 21. DVI (decreased vasculosyncytial membranes). Distal villi show a thickened layer of syncytiotrophoblast, increased villous cytotrophoblast, increased stromal connective tissue, and a paucity of close contacts between capillaries and syncytium (H&E stain, original magnification 20×).

other nutrients to cross the interhemal membrane and hence decrease placental reserve. The pathogenesis is believed to relate to overexpression of placental growth factors, such as insulin and the insulin-like growth factors, leading to villous growth at the expense of terminal differentiation. Accordingly, DVI is most prevalent in placentas from diabetic mothers.[43] Diabetic pregnancies, along with other conditions sharing this placental phenotype, are shown to have an increased incidence of unexplained late stillbirth.[44]

Relation to CNS Injury

An association of DVI with increased susceptibility to CNS injury is not clearly established and is supported mainly by the high prevalence in stillborns. Two small studies, however, have shown a high prevalence in cases of perinatal stroke and a significant relationship to surrogate markers of adverse outcome, such as low Apgar score at 5 and 10 minutes.[21,45]

Pathologic Characteristics

Placental weights with DVI are often outside of the normal limits for gestational age—low when associated with FGR and high when associated with maternal diabetes. Groups with low and high placental weights share a decreased fetoplacental weight ratio, which is used as a surrogate measure for this phenotype. In addition to the histologic characteristics (listed previously), distal villi may

show decreased branching, an edematous or myxoid villous stroma, and, in some cases, excessive proliferation of villous capillaries (either diffuse chorangiosis or multifocal chorangiomatosis).

PERIVILLOUS FIBRIN(OID) DEPOSITION

Definition/Pathogenesis

PVF deposition, in its most severe form, massive PVF deposition or maternal floor infarction, is discussed in the article by Heller elsewhere in this issue. PVF is characterized by an idiopathic accumulation of fibrin and extracellular matrix glycoproteins that completely encircles significant portions of the distal villous tree, preventing access to maternal nutrients. It is related to maternal autoimmune disease, thrombophilic states, and hypertensive disorders, and fetal long-chain 3-hydroxyacyl–coenzyme A dehydrogenase (LCHAD) deficiency.[46–49] Most infants show marked FGR and there are very high rates of perinatal mortality and recurrence in subsequent pregnancies. The composition of the matrix in PVF is similar to that produced by extravillous trophoblast in the basal plate and PVF is commonly associated with large numbers of extravillous trophoblast.

Relation to CNS Injury

Maternal floor infarction is associated with abnormal head ultrasound and a high rate of later neurodevelopmental abnormalities in children of all gestational ages.[50] Lesser degrees of PVF are correlated with CP and other neurodevelopmental disorders in term infants.[34]

Pathologic Characteristics

Gross examination is critical for a diagnosis of massive PVF. Typically, a large portion of the basal plate is thickened by consolidation of adjacent villous parenchyma (usually at least 0.5–2 cm in diameter). Less commonly, patchy consolidation of the entire villous parenchyma is noted. Less than 10% to 20% involvement after a reliable gross examination probably excludes the diagnosis. Histologically, PVF shows 2 patterns, sometimes in different areas of the same placenta (Figs. 22 and 23). In the more rapidly developing pattern, villi are surrounded by bright red fibrin-type fibrinoid with areas of rarefaction, suggesting clot retraction. Extravillous trophoblast is sparse and villi show ischemic changes. In the more slowly evolving form, pink flocculent matrix-type fibrinoid predominates, there are many extravillous trophoblast, and villi show involutional changes.

PITFALLS/DIFFERENTIAL DIAGNOSIS

Some of the lesions typical of MMP, such as decreased placental weight, thin UC, and peripheral UC insertion, may be seen in other conditions, including suboptimal uterine implantation site, chronic maternal disease, maternal steroid therapy, fetal genetic or chromosomal disorders,

and chronic placental inflammation (Box 4). Chorangiomas, maternal leiomyomas and areas of placental atrophy or PVF plaques, like infarcts, present as firm gross lesions. Only PVF plaques and marginal atrophy present diagnostic challenges. Collapse of the intervillous space, karyorrhectic debris, and changes consistent with severe MMP in surrounding villi favor infarcts over the other 2 lesions. With respect to accelerated maturation, cognizance of gestational age, the typical alternating biphasic pattern at low power, other associated pathologic features, and experience are all important for avoiding misdiagnosis.

The most important consideration in the differential diagnosis of DVI is to exclude true prematurity in cases of uncertain gestational age. This is best realized by comparing fetal and placental weights to standard placental growth charts and by having a working familiarity with the normal villous architecture of each gestational age range. A diagnosis of DVI should be made reluctantly in placentas delivered before 37 weeks. Although some placentas with DVI have chorangiosis, a majority of placentas with chorangiosis do not have DVI. Villous edema associated with hydrops may superficially mimic DVI but lacks most of the typical histologic features other than edematous myxoid stroma. Finally, hypercoiling of the UC is associated with DVI, and chronic placental congestion may be a second etiologic factor for DVI.[51] Careful attention should be paid to the other

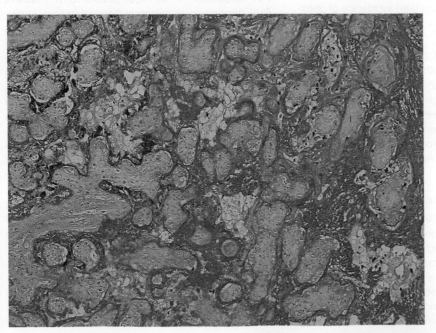

Fig. 22. Massive PVF deposition, rapidly evolving pattern. Villi are completely involuted but, unlike villous infarction, remain separated by hypereosinophilic fibrin-type fibrinoid with scant extravillous trophoblast (H&E stain, original magnification 4×).

Fig. 23. Massive PVF deposition, slowly evolving pattern. Involuted villi are surrounded by pink matrix type-fibrinoid material containing large numbers of extravillous trophoblast (H&E stain, original magnification 4×).

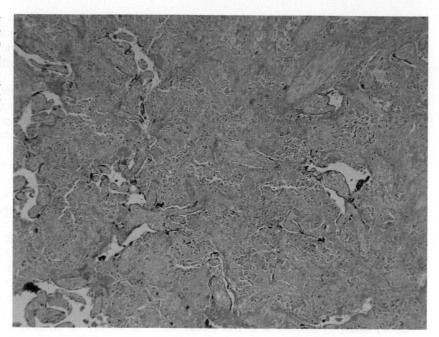

pathologic features of chronic UC compression (discussed previously) before making a diagnosis of isolated DVI.

PVF deposition is distinguished from PVF plaques and placental atrophy by its more diffuse nature. PVF differs from intervillous fibrin seen in MMP by virtue of circumferential involvement of individual villi and incorporation of large numbers of contiguous villi. Clinical history may be helpful because massive PVF is usually accompanied by FGR and often associated with previous pregnancy losses.

Box 4
Uteroplacental insufficiency/decreased placental reserve

Key Features

	Placental Weight	Fetal Weight	Fetoplacental Weight Ratio	Villous Maturity/GA	Villous Agglutination	Local Lesions—IVS Collapsed	Local Lesions—IVS Retained
MMP	↓↓	↓	↑↑	↑	+	++	—
DVI	Variable		↓	↓	—	—	—
Massive PVF	Variable	↓↓	Variable	Variable	++	—	+
PVF plaque(s)	Normal	Normal	Normal	Normal	—	—	++

Abbreviations: GA, gestational age; IVS, intervillous space.

Pitfalls/Differential Diagnosis

Unknown or incorrect GA

Placental atrophy (usually marginal)

PLACENTAL BIOMARKERS

OVERVIEW

An underappreciated concept in perinatal biology is that the placenta is also a rich source of indicators for processes occurring outside its confines. These findings often do not affect placental function but rather serve as biomarkers for understanding the range of physiologic processes affecting a pregnancy. In general, these responses are subdivided into mild, moderate, and severe subgroups. A finding of 1 or more biomarker lesions combined with other placental lesions is highly significant and severe variants of each process may directly contribute to CNS damage.

FETAL INFLAMMATORY RESPONSE TO BACTERIAL INFECTION

Bacterial infections of the amniotic fluid (see the article by Baergen elsewhere in this issue) are associated with ACA and contribute to neurodisability in several ways. ACA can lead to premature delivery with its attendant increased risk for CNS injury. Bacteria can spread to the fetus, causing congenital or early-onset neonatal sepsis, a type of sentinel event with a high rate of death and neurologic complications. Most often, however, infection remains confined to the placenta and bacterial products, known as pathogen-associated molecular patterns (PAMPs) (eg,

lipopolysaccharide), are released, eliciting fetal cytokines and other inflammatory mediators associated with the FIR syndrome, a significant risk factor for CNS injury, particularly in the premature infant.[52]

The maternal and fetal responses to bacterial infection in the amniotic fluid are distinct.[53] Each can be subcategorized in terms of intensity (grade) and duration (stage). There is little evidence that any type of maternal response has an influence on CNS outcomes. The FIR begins in the umbilical vein and chorionic plate vessels (stage 1), progresses to involve the umbilical artery (stage 2), and culminates in the formation of bands of neutrophils surrounding fetal vessels in Wharton jelly (stage 3). Infiltration of the umbilical arteries is shown in 2 studies to predict higher levels of circulating fetal cytokines (**Fig. 24**).[54,55] Funisitis is an ambiguous term usually but not always used to denote involvement of both vessels and Wharton jelly. It is correlated with a variety of adverse outcomes, including CP, interventricular hemorrhage, white matter damage, and developmental delay.[52,56] Near-confluent infiltration of chorionic vessels (grade 2 FIR) is associated with neurologic impairment in premature and term infants (**Fig. 25**).[34,40] Finally, fetal vasculitis promotes the development of chorionic vessel thrombi that are associated with neurodisability in VLBW infants and which can occasionally embolize to the fetal brain, causing perinatal stroke (**Fig. 26**).[40]

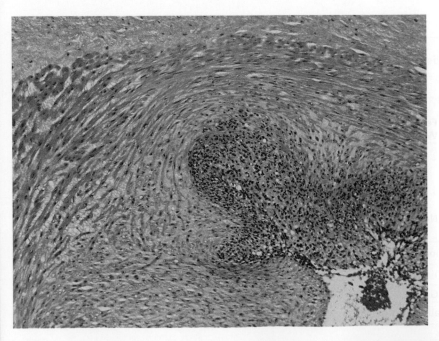

Fig. 24. Umbilical arteritis (ACA, stage 2 FIR). The subintimal layer of the umbilical artery is infiltrated by neutrophils (H&E stain, original magnification 10×).

Fig. 25. Severe acute chorionic vasculitis with vessel wall damage (ACA, grade 2 FIR). The upper muscular wall of a large chorionic vessel shows near-confluent infiltration by neutrophils associated with necrosis and loss of normal architecture (H&E stain, original magnification 20×).

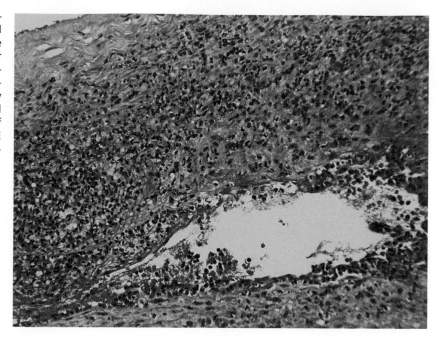

FETAL MECONIUM RELEASE, DURATION OF EXPOSURE

Term and near-term fetuses (greater than 34 weeks) mount a parasympathetic response to acute hypoxia that leads to decreased intestinal perfusion and defecation of meconium into the amniotic fluid. The prevalence of meconium release reaches 30% for deliveries at 41 weeks or more.

Although it is a biomarker for fetal hypoxia, meconium can also exert toxic effects on the placenta by inducing vasospasm and tissue necrosis due to its high levels of bile acids and phospholipases.

Meconium-related changes in the membranes alone (necrosis, edema, and pigment-laden macrophages) are not significantly associated with CNS injury (**Fig. 27**). More prolonged exposure to meconium (greater than 6–12 h), as determined

Fig. 26. Nonocclusive chorionic vessel thrombosis secondary to ACA with fetal vasculitis. The upper muscular wall of a large chorionic vessel shows moderate infiltration by neutrophils and a region of adherent, recent nonocclusive thrombosis (H&E stain, original magnification 4×).

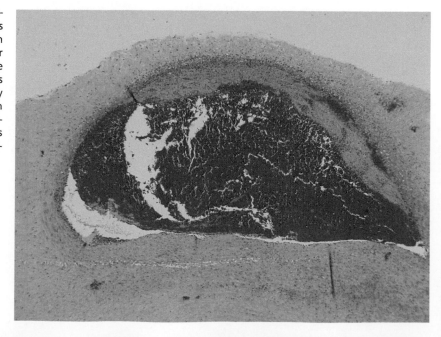

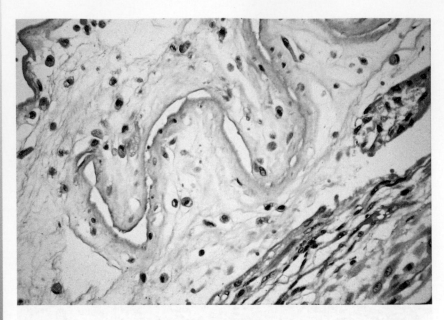

Fig. 27. Recent meconium exposure. Amnion is edematous with mild epithelial degeneration. There are numerous vacuolated, meconium pigment–laden macrophages (H&E stain, original magnification 10×).

by the presence of vacuolated pigment-laden macrophages in the chorionic plate, chorionic vessel walls, and Wharton jelly, predicts a low but significant risk for CNS damage (**Fig. 28**).[18] Least commonly, meconium can trigger apoptosis of vascular smooth muscle cells, a lesion known as meconium associated vascular necrosis

(MAVN).[57,58] Factors increasing the risk of MAVN include intact membranes, oligohydramnios, increased volume of meconium, and prolonged exposure. MAVN is a highly significant risk factor for CP, severe NE with neonatal death, and related forms of long-term neurodisability.[13] Gross features associated with a higher risk of MAVN

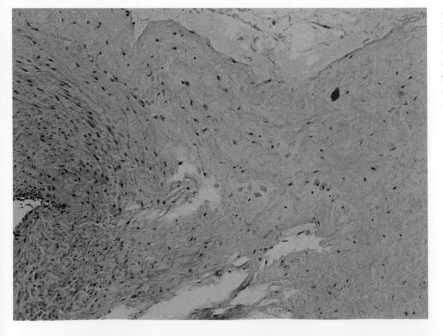

Fig. 28. Prolonged meconium exposure. Pigment-laden, vacuolated macrophages are seen deep in the connective tissue of the chorionic plate (H&E stain, original magnification 4×).

include intense dark-green staining of the entire chorionic sac and UC. Microscopically, MAVN is characterized by rounded, intensely eosinophilic apoptotic bodies with a small central pyknotic nucleus at the periphery of chorionic and occasionally umbilical vessel walls on the side facing the amniotic fluid (**Fig. 29**).

ERYTHROBLASTIC RESPONSE TO REDUCED FETAL OXYGEN TENSION

Increased intramedullary and extramedullary hematopoiesis with premature release of immature nucleated red blood cell precursors (NRBCs) into the peripheral circulation is a well-known adaptive response to decreased fetal oxygen tension.[59] Profound elevations in the NRBC count are seen with severe fetal anemia whereas lesser degrees of elevation are more common with prolonged hypoxia. Identification of increased NRBCs in placental sections is a useful biomarker. As shown in humans and animal models, circulating NRBC accumulate slowly becoming detectable by histologic examination approximately 6 to 12 hours after the onset of the hypoxic stimulus.[60,61] One study comparing the number of NRBCs in placental sections with neonatal blood count showed that a finding of more than 10 NRBCs per 10 high-power field (40×) corresponds to an absolute neonatal NRBC count of greater than 2500/mm^3 (**Fig. 30**).[61] Although NRBCs have no direct role in

causation, their elevation is a risk factor for CNS injury in term infants.[34,62]

PITFALLS/DIFFERENTIAL DIAGNOSIS

The main differential diagnosis of ACA is membrane inflammation related to ischemia (laminar necrosis) or antigenic stimulation (lymphoplasmacytic deciduitis) (**Box 5**). The keys to avoiding overdiagnosis are a strict requirement for neutrophils in subchorionic plate fibrin, diffuse involvement of membranes, and localization in chorion, rather than exclusively decidua.

Conditions mimicking meconium-related changes are separated into 2 groups: those associated with green staining and those associated with pigment-laden macrophages. Chronic abruption (biliverdin staining) and severe ACA (green purulent exudates) cause green staining. Hemosiderin and nonspecific lipofuschin are other pigments seen in macrophages. The keys to specific diagnosis are term or near-term gestation, clinical history of meconium-stained fluid, toxic effects in the amnion, and typical vacuolated macrophages with a fine dusty, brown-red pigment. The differential diagnosis of MAVN includes vascular degenerative changes seen in the UC of macerated stillborns-nonspecific cytoplasmic eosinophilia lacking typical changes of apoptosis (described in this discussion).

The differential diagnosis of hypoxia-related elevation of NRBCs includes clusters of NRBCs or

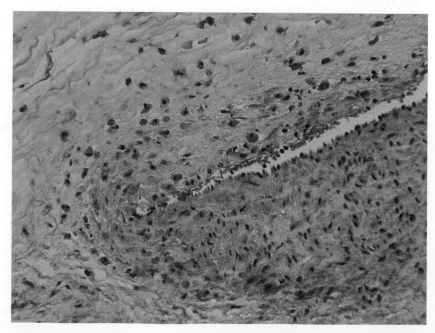

Fig. 29. MAVN. Superficial myocytes in upper wall of a large chorionic vessel show apoptotic changes including rounded contour, intense cytoplasmic eosinophilia, and nuclear pyknosis (H&E stain, original magnification 20×).

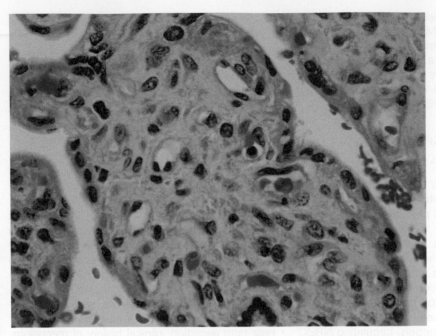

Fig. 30. Increased circulating fetal NRBCs (H&E stain, original magnification 60×). A mononuclear cell within one of the villous capillaries shows diagnostic features of erythroid lineage (perfectly round nucleus with hyperchromasia and featureless nuclear chromatin plus glassy eosinophilic cytoplasm).

erythroblasts in villous capillaries, which are more common with fetal anemia or blood loss, and other mononuclear cells that mimic NRBCs. Lymphocytes are also transiently elevated with hypoxia. Myelomonocytic cells may be increased in transient myeloproliferative disorder seen in some cases of trisomy 21. Adherence to strict diagnostic criteria, such as round nuclei, hyperchromatic featureless chromatin, and glassy eosinophilic cytoplasm, should prevent misdiagnosis.

Box 5
Biomarker lesions

Acute chorioamnionitis

Key Features

　　Neutrophils in subchorionic fibrin (chorionic plate)

　　Diffuse involvement of choridecidual interface (membranes)

Pitfalls/Differential Diagnosis

　　Laminar necrosis of membranes

　　Lymphoplasmacytic deciduitis

　　Degenerative nuclear changes in umbilical myocytes (pseudovasculitis)

　　Chronic fetal vasculitis (see section: placental syndromes: fetal vasculopathies)

Meconium-related changes

Key Features

　　Clinical history

　　Green staining

　　Edematous slippery membranes

　　Vacuolated macrophages (with pigment)

Pitfalls/Differential Diagnosis

　　Other green placentas (chronic abruption and severe chorioamnionitis)

　　Other macrophage pigments (hemosiderin and lipofuschin)

　　Other causes of membrane edema (prolonged rupture of membranes, hydrops, and gastroschisis)

SYNTHESIS OF PLACENTAL FINDINGS AND NEUROLOGIC OUTCOME

The first priority in relating placental findings to outcome is to consider how they fit in with and supplement the clinical facts of a case. Some placental lesions may be so unambiguous as to stand alone regardless of the clinical history. Others are context dependent and must be judged as to severity, specificity, and the confidence with which they are made. For example, care should be taken before diagnosing

- Abruption placenta in a case without evidence of Vaginal bleeding
- Fetal hemorrhage in the absence of fetal shock or anemia
- MAVN without meconium-stained fluid
- MMP in the face of normal fetal and placental weights
- DVI in an infant of uncertain gestational age

This article has necessarily focused on individual lesions. However, in virtually every study in which they were assessed, the finding of multiple independent placental lesions is a stronger risk factor for CNS injury than any individual lesion.[19,34] Synergy is demonstrated with each additional placental finding, and some evidence suggests that lesions occurring at different times have a greater affect than those occurring at the same time. Even in cases of a documented sentinel event, studies have found a high prevalence of additional placental lesions that may have played a role in the eventual outcome.[29]

A key question in cases of CNS injury is timing, and it is not uncommon for clinicians, risk managers, and lawyers to ask a pathologist to estimate how long a lesion has been present. This is best accomplished by considering the results of experimental studies, by analogy to similar processes in other organ systems, and by personal experience with similar cases where timing is well established. A classification scheme that I use is to separate lesions into chronic (weeks in duration), subacute (more than 6–12 h), less than 1 week, and acute (fewer than 6–12 h) subgroups. Any further precision is probably unwarranted. A listing of the lesions discussed in this article in terms of this scheme is shown in **Table 2**.

The final and most important consideration is how far to go when asked whether the placental pathology caused the adverse clinical outcome. First, it needs to be emphasized that there is never a one-to-one correspondence between lesions observed in the placenta and the integrity of the fetal brain. Every placental lesion, no matter how

Table 2
Approximate timing of placental findings

Acute (less than 6–12 h)	Abruptio placenta Complete UC occlusion Fetal vessel lacerations ACA without FIR Recent meconium exposure (membrane necrosis/pigment) FMH (most)
Subacute (6–12 h to 1 wk)	Subacute abruption Fetal thrombotic vasculopathy, villous stromal vascular karyorrhexis ACA with FIR Prolonged meconium exposure (chorionic pate pigment, MAVN) Chronic/partial intermittent UC compression (most) FMH (some)
Chronic (more than 1 wk)	Fetal thrombotic vasculopathy, avascular villi Chronic villitis (VUE) ± OFV Chronic abruption/peripheral separation MMP PVF deposition DVI Chronic/partial intermittent UC compression (some) FMH (rare)

severe, has been found in fetuses without CNS injury and many cases of neurodisability have no identifiable placental lesions. The pertinent questions are

1. Is the lesion sufficient to cause brain injury?
2. What is the strength of the association?
3. Considering the entire clinicopathologic picture, what are the chances that the child would have escaped an adverse outcome in the absence of the placental findings?

A useful analogy is an autopsy performed on a 45-year-old man who drops dead walking down the street. Autopsy reveals a myocardial infarction. Although many individuals survive such a lesion, it is capable of causing sudden death and, in the absence of other causative factors, is likely to have been the cause of death without which the individual would still be alive.

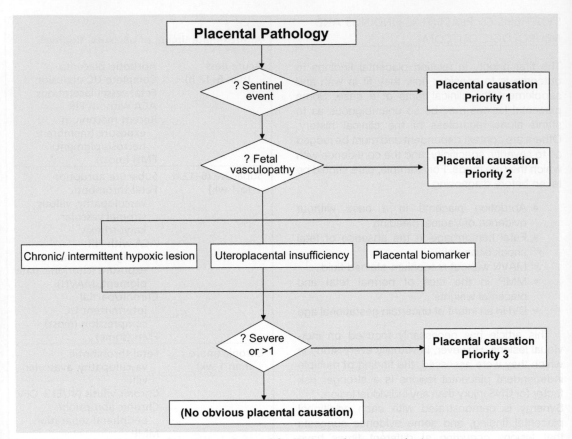

Fig. 31. Hierarchical algorithm for relating placental findings to adverse neurologic outcome.

An algorithm illustrating a hierarchical approach to assigning placental causation in terms of the lesions and biomarkers discussed in this article is provided in **Fig. 31.**

REFERENCES

1. Himmelmann K, Hagberg G, Uvebrant P. The changing panorama of cerebral palsy in Sweden. X. Prevalence and origin in the birth-year period 1999-2002. Acta Paediatr 2010;99(9):1337–43.

2. Myers RE. Two patterns of perinatal brain damage and their conditions of occurrence. Am J Obstet Gynecol 1972;112:246–76.

3. Martinez-Biarge M, Madero R, Gonzalez A, et al. Perinatal morbidity and risk of hypoxic-ischemic encephalopathy associated with intrapartum sentinel events. Am J Obstet Gynecol 2012;206(2): 148.e1–7.

4. Hankins GD, Koen S, Gei AF, et al. Neonatal organ system injury in acute birth asphyxia sufficient to result in neonatal encephalopathy. Obstet Gynecol 2002;99(5 Pt 1):688–91.

5. Badawi N, Felix JF, Kurinczuk JJ, et al. Cerebral palsy following term newborn encephalopathy: a population-based study. Dev Med Child Neurol 2005;47(5):293–8.

6. Parast MM, Crum CP, Boyd TK. Placental histologic criteria for umbilical blood flow restriction in unexplained stillbirth. Hum Pathol 2008;39(6):948–53.

7. Martin GC, Green RS, Holzman IR. Acidosis in newborns with nuchal cords and normal Apgar scores. J Perinatol 2005;25(3):162–5.

8. Stroustrup A, Trasande L. Demographics, clinical characteristics and outcomes of neonates diagnosed with fetomaternal haemorrhage. Arch Dis Child Fetal Neonatal Ed 2012;97:F405–10.

9. Kaplan C, Blanc WA, Elias J. Identification of erythrocytes in intervillous thrombi: a study using immunoperoxidase identification of hemoglobins. Hum Pathol 1982;13:554–7.

10. Fox H. Pathology of the placenta. 2nd edition. London: W. B. Saunders; 1997.

11. Redline RW, Pappin A. Fetal thrombotic vasculopathy: the clinical significance of extensive avascular villi. Hum Pathol 1995;26:80–5.

12. McDonald DG, Kelehan P, McMenamin JB, et al. Placental fetal thrombotic vasculopathy is associated with neonatal encephalopathy. Hum Pathol 2004;35(7):875–80.

13. Redline RW. Severe fetal placental vascular lesions in term infants with neurologic impairment. Am J Obstet Gynecol 2005;192:452–7.

14. Xiao W, Mindrinos MN, Seok J, et al. A genomic storm in critically injured humans. J Exp Med 2011; 208(13):2581–90.

15. Vern TZ, Alles AJ, KowalVern A, et al. Frequency of factor V-Leiden and prothrombin G20210A in placentas and their relationship with placental lesions. Hum Pathol 2000;31(9):1036–43.

16. Redline RW. Clinical and pathological umbilical cord abnormalities in fetal thrombotic vasculopathy. Hum Pathol 2004;35(12):1494–8.

17. Chang KT, Keating S, Costa S, et al. Third-trimester stillbirths: correlative neuropathology and placental pathology. Pediatr Dev Pathol 2011;14(5):345–52.

18. Wintermark P, Boyd T, Gregas MC, et al. Placental pathology in asphyxiated newborns meeting the criteria for therapeutic hypothermia. Am J Obstet Gynecol 2010;203(6):579.e1–9.

19. Viscardi RM, Sun CC. Placental lesion multiplicity: risk factor for IUGR and neonatal cranial ultrasound abnormalities. Early Hum Dev 2001;62(1):1–10.

20. Chisholm KM, Heerema-McKenney A, Tian L, et al. Correlation of preterm infant morbidities with placenta histology. Mod Pathol 2012;25:323.

21. Elbers J, Viero S, MacGregor D, et al. Placental pathology in neonatal stroke. Pediatrics 2011; 127(3):e722–9.

22. Redline RW, Ariel I, Baergen RN, et al. Fetal vascular obstructive lesions: nosology and reproducibility of placental reaction patterns. Pediatr Dev Pathol 2004;7:443–52.

23. Redline RW. Villitis of unknown etiology: noninfectious chronic villitis in the placenta. Hum Pathol 2007;38(10):1439–46.

24. Scher MS, Trucco GS, Beggarly ME, et al. Neonates with electrically confirmed seizures and possible placental associations. Pediatr Neurol 1998;19:37–41.

25. Jacques SM, Qureshi F, Kim CJ, et al. Eosinophilic/T-cell chorionic vasculitis: a clinicopathologic and immunohistochemical study of 51 cases. Pediatr Dev Pathol 2011;14(3):198–205.

26. Frasch MG, Mansano RZ, McPhaul L, et al. Measures of acidosis with repetitive umbilical cord occlusions leading to fetal asphyxia in the near-term ovine fetus. Am J Obstet Gynecol 2009;200(2):200.e1–7.

27. Clapp JF 3rd, Lopez B, Simonean S. Nuchal cord and neurodevelopmental performance at 1 year. J Soc Gynecol Investig 1999;6(5):268–72.

28. Grafe MR. The correlation of prenatal brain damage with placental pathology. J Neuropathol Exp Neurol 1994;53:407–15.

29. Redline RW. Cerebral palsy in term infants: a clinicopathologic analysis of 158 medicolegal case reviews. Pediatr Dev Pathol 2008;11(6):456–64.

30. Gruenwald P, Levin H, Yousem H. Abruption and premature separation of the placenta. The clinical and pathologic entity. Am J Obstet Gynecol 1968; 102:604–10.

31. Harris BA. Peripheral placental separation: a review. Obstet Gynecol Surv 1988;43:577–81.

32. Naftolin F, Khudr G, Benirschke K, et al. The syndrome of chronic abruptio placentae, hydrorrhea, and circumallate placenta. Am J Obstet Gynecol 1973;116:347–50.

33. Nelson KB, Ellenberg JH. Obstetric complications as risk factors for cerebral palsy or seizure disorders. JAMA 1984;251:1843–8.

34. Redline RW, O'Riordan MA. Placental lesions associated with cerebral palsy and neurologic impairment following term birth. Arch Pathol Lab Med 2000; 124(12):1785–91.

35. Redline RW, Wilson-Costello D. Chronic peripheral separation of placenta: the significance of diffuse chorioamnionic hemosiderosis. Am J Clin Pathol 1999;111:804–10.

36. Redline RW, Boyd T, Campbell V, et al. Maternal vascular underperfusion: nosology and reproducibility of placental reaction patterns. Pediatr Dev Pathol 2004;7:237–49.

37. Pijnenborg R. The placental bed. Hypertens Pregnancy 1996;15:7–23.

38. Burke CJ, Tannenberg AE. Prenatal brain damage and placental infarction: an autopsy study. Dev Med Child Neurol 1995;37:555–62.

39. Blair E, de Groot J, Nelson KB. Placental infarction identified by macroscopic examination and risk of cerebral palsy in infants at 35 weeks of gestational age and over. Am J Obstet Gynecol 2011;205(2): 124.e1–7.

40. Redline RW, Wilson-Costello D, Borawski E, et al. Placental lesions associated with neurologic impairment and cerebral palsy in very low birth weight infants. Arch Pathol Lab Med 1998;122: 1091–8.

41. Kumazaki K, Nakayama M, Sumida Y, et al. Placental features in preterm infants with periventricular leukomalacia. Pediatrics 2002;109(4):650–5.

42. Redlline RW. Distal villous immaturity. Diagn Histopathol 2012;18(5):189–94.

43. Driscoll SG. The pathology of pregnancy complicated by diabetes mellitus. Med Clin North Am 1965;49:1053–65.

44. Stallmach T, Hebisch G, Meier K, et al. Rescue by birth: defective placental maturation and late fetal mortality. Obstet Gynecol 2001;97(4):505–9.

45. Shehata F, Levin I, Shrim A, et al. Placenta/birthweight ratio and perinatal outcome: a retrospective cohort analysis. BJOG 2011;118(6):741–7.

46. Andres RL, Kuyper W, Resnik R, et al. The association of maternal floor infarction of the placenta with adverse perinatal outcome. Am J Obstet Gynecol 1990;163:935–8.

47. Bendon RW, Hommel AB. Maternal floor infarction in autoimmune disease: two cases. Pediatr Pathol Lab Med 1996;16:293–7.

48. Katz VL, DiTomasso J, Farmer R, et al. Activated protein C resistance associated with maternal floor infarction treated with low-molecular-weight heparin. Am J Perinatol 2002;19(5):273–7.

49. Matern D, Schehata BM, Shekhawa P, et al. Placental floor infarction complicating the pregnancy of a fetus with long-chain 3-hydroxyacyl-CoA dehydrogenase (LCHAD) deficiency. Mol Genet Metab 2001;72(3):265–8.

50. Adams-Chapman I, Vaucher YE, Bejar RF, et al. Maternal floor infarction of the placenta: association with central nervous system injury and adverse neurodevelopmental outcome. J Perinatol 2002;22(3):236–41.

51. de Laat MW, van der Meij JJ, Visser GH, et al. Hypercoiling of the umbilical cord and placental maturation defect: associated pathology? Pediatr Dev Pathol 2007;10(4):293–9.

52. Mittendorf R, Montag AG, MacMillan W, et al. Components of the systemic fetal inflammatory response syndrome as predictors of impaired neurologic outcomes in children. Am J Obstet Gynecol 2003;188(6):1438–44.

53. Redline R, Faye-Petersen O, Heller D, et al. Amniotic infection syndrome: nosology and reproducibility of placental reaction patterns. Pediatr Dev Pathol 2003;6:445–58.

54. Kim CJ, Yoon BH, Romero R, et al. Umbilical arteritis and phlebitis mark different stages of the fetal inflammatory response. Am J Obstet Gynecol 2001;185(2):496–500.

55. Rogers BB, Alexander JM, Head J, et al. Umbilical vein interleukin-6 levels correlate with the severity of placental inflammation and gestational age. Hum Pathol 2002;33(3):335–40.

56. Leviton A, Paneth N, Reuss ML, et al. Maternal infection, fetal inflammatory response, and brain damage in very low birth weight infants. Developmental Epidemiology Network Investigators. Pediatr Res 1999;46(5):566–75.

57. Altshuler G, Arizawa M, Molnar-Nadasdy G. Meconium-induced umbilical cord vascular necrosis and ulceration: a potential link between the placenta and poor pregnancy outcome. Obstet Gynecol 1992;79:760–6.

58. Redline RW. Meconium associated vascular necrosis. Pathol Case Rev 2010;15(3):55–7.

59. Hermansen MC. Nucleated red blood cells in the fetus and newborn. Arch Dis Child Fetal Neonatal Ed 2001;84(3):F211–5.

60. Blackwell SC, Hallak M, Hotra JW, et al. Timing of fetal nucleated red blood cell count elevation in response to acute hypoxia. Biol Neonate 2004;85(4):217–20.

61. Redline RW. Elevated circulating fetal nucleated red blood cells and placental pathology in term infants who develop cerebral palsy. Hum Pathol 2008;39(9):1378–84.

62. Phelan JP, Korst LM, Ahn MO, et al. Neonatal nucleated red blood cell and lymphocyte counts in fetal brain injury. Obstet Gynecol 1998;91(4):485–9.

Placenta Accreta and Percreta

Debra S. Heller, MD*

KEYWORDS

- Placenta accreta • Placenta increta • Placenta percreta • Uterus (pathology) • Pregnancy
- Myometrium (pathology) • Hysterectomy

ABSTRACT

The incidence of abnormally adherent placenta (accreta/percreta) has increased 10-fold in the past 50 years, predominantly due to the increased use of cesarean section delivery. The causes, clinical correlates, and pathology of these conditions are discussed in this article.

OVERVIEW

Placenta accreta is defined as the abnormal adherence of the placenta to the wall of the uterus.[1] Abnormally adherent placenta is traditionally divided into accreta for placentas implanted onto the myometrium without underlying decidua, increta for those invading myometrium, and percreta for those penetrating the entire uterine wall. The term, *creta*, or just *accreta*, is seen in some of the literature, to encompass the entire range of abnormally adherent placentas. The incidence of placenta accreta is estimated to have increased 10 times in the past 50 years, occurring in 1 in 2500 pregnancies,[1] according to some investigators, and in as many as 1 in 533 deliveries, or 9.3% of women with placenta previa.[2] Abnormally adherent placentas are a major source of maternal morbidity and mortality, predominantly related to intrapartum hemorrhage, with risks, including massive transfusion; disseminated intravascular coagulation; infection; uterine rupture with potential fetal death; injury of adjacent organs, particularly genitourinary; formation of fistulas; and death.[2,3] In addition, placenta accreta has been associated with small for gestational age infants and preterm deliveries.[1]

Placenta accreta/percreta now exceeds uterine atony as the main cause of cesarean hysterectomy.[3] It is likely that the incidence is underestimated, because clinically diagnosed cases of retained placenta or need for manual removal of the placenta may reflect lesser degrees of accreta. Women with a prior retained placenta are at increased risk of recurrent retained placenta during subsequent pregnancies,[4] consistent with a focal accreta.

The rising incidence of placenta accreta/percreta has been attributed to the rising use of cesarean section delivery. The use of cesarean delivery in the United States has increased from 5.8% in 1970 to 32.3% in 2008, with an overall increased rate of 50% since 1996.[5] Associated with this increase in cesarean deliveries has been an overall increase in maternal morbidity and mortality, with hemorrhagic complications of placenta accreta associated with multiple uterine scars from multiple cesarean sections contributing to the rise. Placenta accreta associated with multiple cesarean sections has led to a markedly increased rate of peripartum hysterectomies,[5] and the risk goes up with each additional cesarean section a woman undergoes.[6] The origin of accreta after cesarean includes a defect in the decidua basalis as well as abnormal repair and vascularization.[7] Some investigators have also suggested that accreta is more common when a single layer closure is used during previous cesarean sections. Other risk factors for placenta accreta include abnormal placental location, such as placenta previa; prior curettage; number of curettages; myomectomy; advanced maternal age with delayed childbearing; high parity; cornual pregnancy; placenta membranacea, submucosal leiomyomata; and uterine anomalies.[1,3,8] It has been suggested that in vitro

Disclosure: None.

Department of Pathology & Laboratory Medicine, University of Medicine and Dentistry of New Jersey-New Jersey Medical School, 185 South Orange Avenue, Newark, NJ 07103, USA

* Department of Pathology-UH/E158, University of Medicine and Dentistry of New Jersey-New Jersey Medical School, 185 South Orange Avenue, Newark, NJ 07103.

E-mail address: hellerds@umdnj.edu

Surgical Pathology 6 (2013) 181–197
http://dx.doi.org/10.1016/j.path.2012.10.003

Fig. 1. Normal second-trimester implantation site showing placental site giant cells (multinucleated intermediate or extravillous trophoblast) in decidua and myometrium (hematoxylin-eosin).

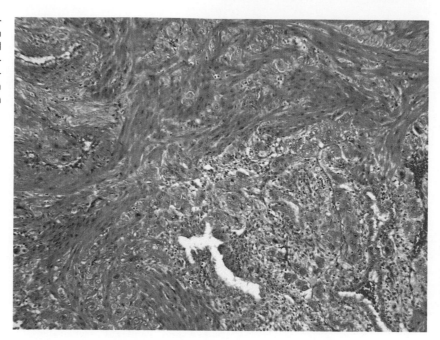

vitro, and Garmi and colleagues postulated a role for careful repair after cesarean sections.

Not all investigators believe increased invasiveness of the placenta is the cause of placenta accreta. The immunohistochemical profile of the extravillous trophoblast has been shown to be the same as in normal gestation.[20] Earl and colleagues suggested that absence of decidua is of importance and that accreta does not seem to arise from increased invasiveness of trophoblast. This viewpoint is further supported by the work of Kim and colleagues,[21] who demonstrated an increased number of CD146-positive implantation site intermediate trophoblasts, in placenta creta (not further subdivided), but did not show any difference in Ki-67, Bcl-2, or cleaved caspase from normal pregnancy. They reported an overlap with exaggerated placental site and placenta creta, with exuberant infiltration of intermediate trophoblasts into the myometrium (**Fig. 2**), as opposed to the occasional scattered ones in normal pregnancy. Also militating against increased trophoblast invasiveness is the study of Li and colleagues,[22] who studied the immunohistochemical staining of the cell adhesion molecules E-cadherin and β-catenin in the villous trophoblast of normal pregnancies and placenta accreta and found no difference.

The most commonly held theory of accreta is that it is due to deficiency of the decidua. This is believed a result of uterine injury or trauma in most cases attributable to uterine surgery, in particular cesarean section delivery. Myometrial fragments are commonly seen after suction or sharp curettage

for abortions, but their relationship to subsequent accreta is unclear. The finding of myometrium curetted out during evacuation of products of conception has not been shown predictive of future accreta, although a past history of termination or miscarriage was found more common in women who required manual removal of the placenta[23] in a series of women with after vaginal delivery. Myometrial tissue was found in the prior specimens of both the women requiring manual removal of the placenta and the controls in this series.

It has been suggested that a subset of accreta may have a genetic origin, based on history of repeat accreta, prior manual removal of placenta in an antecedent pregnancy, or accreta in a primiparous pregnancy.[24]

Tantbirojn and colleagues[3] postulated that placenta creta is multifactorial. They found a decrease in remodeled maternal vessels but deeper vascular remodeling in the myometrium in cases as well as greater depth of extravillous trophoblast invasion. They suggested that greater degrees of creta (ie, increta and percreta) were not from increased invasion by villi but dehiscence of a scar allowing greater penetration of placental tissue.

CLINICAL ASPECTS OF PLACENTA ACCRETA/PERCRETA

CLINICAL DIAGNOSIS

Although most accreta presents in the third trimester as intrapartum hemorrhage, accreta

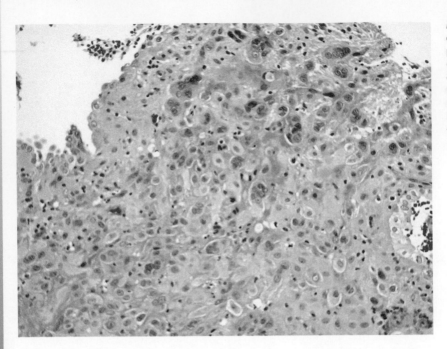

Fig. 2. Exaggerated placental site. Numerous placental site giant cells (multinucleated intermediate or extravillous trophoblast) and single nucleated intermediate trophoblast invading decidua (hematoxylin-eosin).

may be clinically apparent earlier in gestation or before delivery. Second-trimester cases, as well as some third-trimester cases, may present with antepartum hemorrhage or uterine perforation or rupture.[25] Second-trimester cases may also present as postabortal hemorrhage. Rashbaum and colleagues,[26] in a large series of second-trimester dilatation and evacuation cases, found a 0.04% rate of accreta, associated with prior cesarean section and placenta previa. First-trimester presentation is rare. The earliest documented case of increta was reportedly at 5 weeks from last menstrual period in a patient who had a hysterectomy for massive bleeding after curettage for missed abortion. Her prior history was positive for a cesarean section, a vaginal birth after cesarean delivery, and then a curettage for a first-trimester spontaneous abortion.[27]

The bladder is the most common organ involved outside the uterus in placenta percreta.[28] Predelivery hematuria is not a reliable sign nor is cystoscopy reliable in predelivery diagnosis.[29] Urologic complications are high, and someone with urologic expertise should be involved in the planning and care of the patient.

Although most hemorrhage occurs in the intrapartum period after delivery of an infant, delayed heavy bleeding due to persistent creta has also been described. In Walter and colleagues'[30] case, the patient presented 17 weeks after evacuation of an 11-week missed abortion. She had a prior history of cesarean section.

Diagnosis before delivery can allow for treatment planning, which may include a planned hysterectomy or more conservative therapy. In a study of 99 consecutive cases of accreta conducted by Warshak and colleagues,[31] those diagnosed before delivery received fewer units of packed red cells and had a lower estimated blood loss. Overall, planned delivery at 34 to 35 weeks did not significantly increase neonatal morbidity in this cohort.

To diagnose placenta accreta antenatally, it needs to be suspected. Placenta creta can be associated with elevated maternal serum α-fetoprotein and free β–human chorionic gonadotropin[22,32] but not in all cases.[32,33] It has also been suggested that an unexplained second-trimester elevation in maternal serum α-fetoprotein or free β–human chorionic gonadotropin levels may be associated with increased risk of creta.

ULTRASOUND AND MRI FINDINGS IN PLACENTA ACCRETA/PERCRETA AND THEIR ACCURACY

If a patient is considered at risk for a placenta creta, ultrasound or MRI has been used to make an antepartum diagnosis, because advance planning is helpful to minimize morbidity.[28] Although it has been possible in some cases, ultrasound diagnosis of placenta creta in the first trimester is not reliable.[25]

Ultrasonographic findings associated with placenta creta include presence of irregularly shaped vascular spaces within the placenta (lacunae); thinning of the myometrium over the placenta; loss or thinning of the retroplacental clear space or hypoechoic zone that separates myometrium from placenta; thinning, irregularity, or disruption of the linear hyperechoic uterine serosa/bladder interface; protrusion of the placenta into the bladder or mass-like elevations or extensions of tissue with the same echogenicity of placenta beyond the uterine serosa; increased vascularity of the uterine serosa/bladder interface (**Fig. 3**); and turbulent blood flow through placental vascular spaces with Doppler.[28,34,35] These likely result in the increased intervillous thrombi seen in the placentas in cases of placenta accreta. Ultrasound is as sensitive as MRI in most cases of accreta, except in cases of posterior accreta, where MRI may be more useful.[28]

In a retrospective study of antepartum diagnosis,[2] patients with a history of placenta previa, low-lying placenta with prior cesarean section, or prior myomectomy, ultrasound was found to have 0.77 sensitivity and 0.96 specificity for diagnosing accreta. When subsequent MRI was performed on some of their patients with inconclusive findings, the sensitivity was 0.88 and specificity 1.0. Warshak and colleagues[31] recommended ultrasonography as a first investigation, with additional MRI in inconclusive cases to optimize diagnostic accuracy for patients at risk of accreta.

THERAPY FOR ACCRETA

If placenta accreta is not anticipated, a great deal of intrapartum bleeding may be encountered as spontaneous separation occurs or manual separation is attempted, unless the accreta is total. Uteri may be packed, with the placenta sometimes left in place to resorb. This uterine packing risks subsequent delayed and severe infection.[36] Most cases of accreta, increta, and percreta, particularly if unanticipated, have historically come to hysterectomy at the time of delivery. Davis and Cruz[37] reported a case of presumed accreta treated conservatively, which came to hysterectomy 6 months postpartum for persistent intrauterine mass found to be placenta increta.

More recently, efforts at conservative therapy with preservation of the uterus and fertility have included a multidisciplinary approach, which has included hemostatic sutures for focal accreta; uterine wedge resection; leaving the placenta or part of it in situ, placental avoiding uterine incision; intrauterine foley catheter; methotrexate; uterotonics, including intracervical injections of oxytocin, ergometrin, or prostaglandins; interventional radiological procedures, such as arterial balloons or uterine artery embolization; uterine or internal iliac artery ligation; and control of and support for massive hemorrhage.[25,28,38]

FUTURE DIRECTIONS

Although the mainstay of prenatal diagnosis has rested on appropriate suspicion coupled with imaging techniques, it is possible that molecular markers may be available in the future to contribute to the antepartum diagnosis of placenta creta. Mazouni and colleagues[39] describe the technique and appeal of biologic markers in

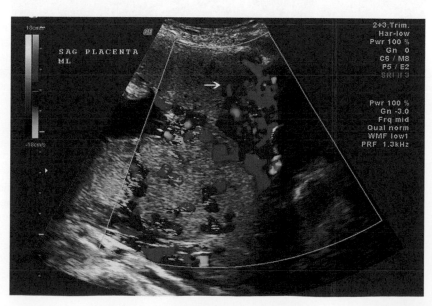

Fig. 3. Placenta previa accreta. Ultrasound image of total previa (U-shaped placenta). The bladder is to the right. Note the marked increase in vascularity (*arrow*), indicating accreta. (*Courtesy of* Abdulla Al-Khan, MD, Hackensack, NJ.)

maternal blood and other molecular markers that can aid the diagnosis of placental abnormalities, including possibly creta. These markers include cell-free fetal DNA, placental mRNA, and DNA microarray. Cell-free placental RNA may be useful in increasing the sensitivity of imaging, as demonstrated by the study of El Behery and colleagues.[40] Future studies for diagnostic utility and cost-benefit analysis are needed before these modalities can be considered for screening.

PATHOLOGIC DIAGNOSIS OF PLACENTA ACCRETA/PERCRETA

The gross appearance of placenta accreta is variable. Placenta accreta may be total; partial, involving one or a few cotyledons; or focal,

involving less than a cotyledon. If the placenta alone is received by a pathology laboratory, there may be no grossly abnormal findings. Alternatively, an area of deficient placental parenchyma may be seen or an area with tightly adherent myometrium. In the case of a hysterectomy when the placenta has been removed manually, the area of accreta may appear shaggier than the rest of the endometrial lining. Adherent placental tissue fragments may be seen in some cases. If the placenta has been left in situ, particularly if it is a complete accreta, the placenta may be seen in situ and is often located in the lower uterine segment anteriorly near a prior cesarean scar or located as a low-lying total or partial placenta previa (**Fig. 4**). Placenta increta may or may not grossly look any different from accreta, although placental tissue

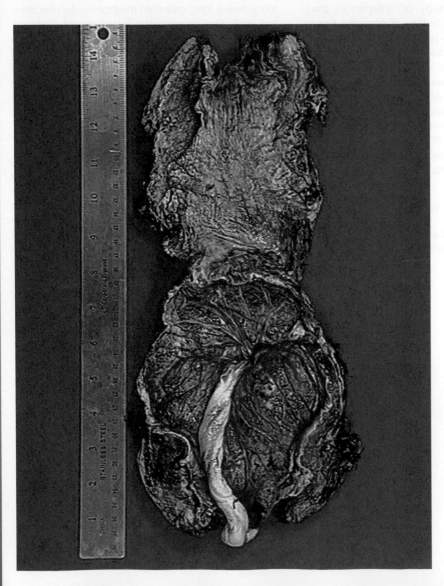

Fig. 4. Total placenta accreta with placenta in situ.

may at times be seen extending into myometrium. The myometrium may be thinned in the area of accreta or increta. Placenta percreta may be obvious, with or without the presence of uterine rupture, and placental tissue may be seen fungating through the defect (**Figs. 5–7**). Percreta may also be more subtle, with marked thinning of the myometrium and a paper-thin grossly membranous tissue confining the placenta. This grossly membranous tissue may represent the uterine serosa or may actually represent the basal plate of the placenta. Applying ink to the area before sectioning may be helpful in interpretation of the slides. The thinned-out area is fragile and may rupture with handling, further complicating diagnosis.

MICROSCOPIC DIAGNOSIS

Normally, at the time of delivery, the placenta separates by cleavage through the decidua basalis (**Fig. 8**) via a shearing action of the uterus contracting and the placenta remaining uncontracted.[8] As an indication of the importance of the presence of decidua, Baergen[8] makes the analogy of tubal ectopic pregnancy, as an example of a tubal percreta due to absent decidua, leading to increased invasiveness and tubal rupture. In placenta accreta, there is a deficiency of the decidua. Placenta accreta may be histologically confirmed on either a hysterectomy specimen (**Figs. 9–11**) or sometimes may be detectable on placental examination (**Fig. 12**). If the placental tissue invades into the

Fig. 5. Placenta percreta with rupture.

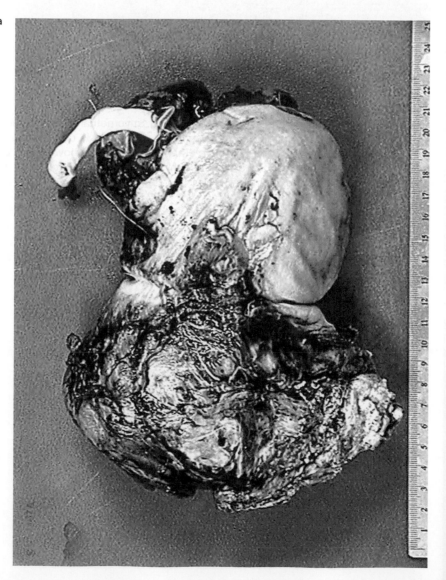

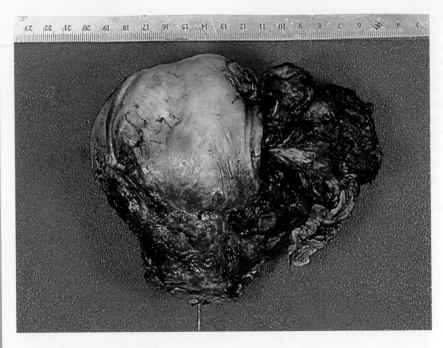

Fig. 6. Placenta percreta with rupture.

myometrium, placenta increta is confirmed (**Figs. 13** and **14**), and if it goes entirely through, percreta can be diagnosed (**Figs. 15** and **16**). Increta and percreta can only be diagnosed on a hysterectomy specimen, not a placental specimen. The finding of myometrial fibers on the maternal surface of the placenta is corroborative of a clinical impression of accreta; however, occasionally fibers can also be found where there is no clinical picture of accreta.[41]

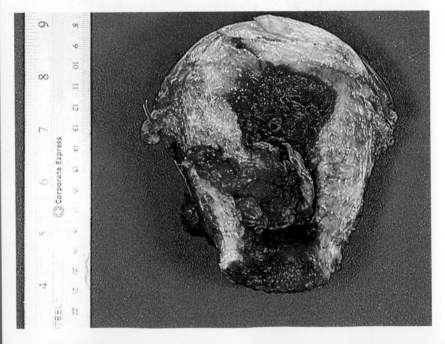

Fig. 7. Cut surface of placenta percreta, showing placental tissue extending through the uterine wall.

Fig. 8. Normal implantation site showing villi in contact with decidua. Myometrium is seen in the upper right (hematoxylin-eosin).

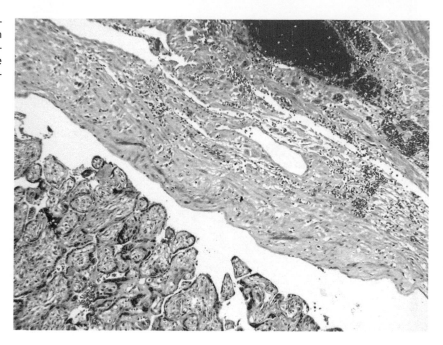

The normal implantation site is comprised of the placenta in contact with basal decidua, which is on the surface of the myometrium in the uterine cavity. The contracting uterine wall after delivery leads to shearing off of the placenta, generally splitting the decidua into the portion adherent to the placenta and a portion remaining lining the endometrial cavity. There are implantation-site intermediate trophoblasts seen in both the decidua and the myometrium, which may resemble exaggerated placental site (**Table 1**). In placenta accreta, there is no intervening

Fig. 9. Placenta accreta—villi in contact with abundant Nitabuch fibrin (hematoxylin-eosin).

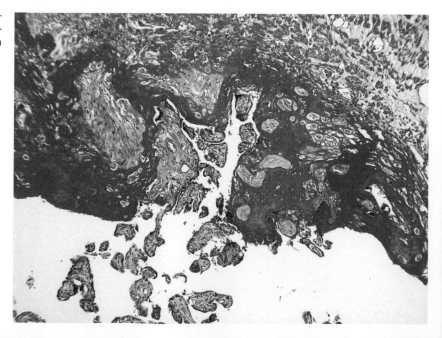

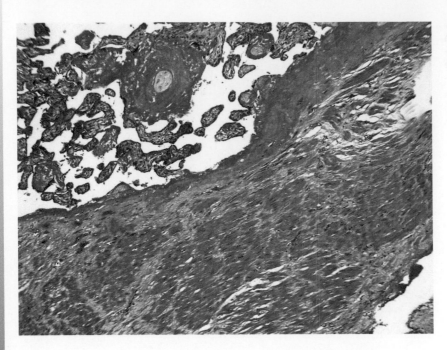

Fig. 10. Placenta accreta—villi in contact with myometrium (hematoxylin-eosin).

decidua, and chorionic villi may be seen in direct apposition to myometrium. This is not as straightforward a diagnosis as it might seem. The interface between placenta and myometrium is irregular to begin with, and a pathologist often receives a disrupted specimen where clinical attempts at manual and surgical removal may have occurred. There is usually an abundant layer of fibrinoid material, the Nitabuch layer, between the placenta and the myometrium, further complicating the interpretation. It is sometimes difficult to distinguish the nonvillous intermediate

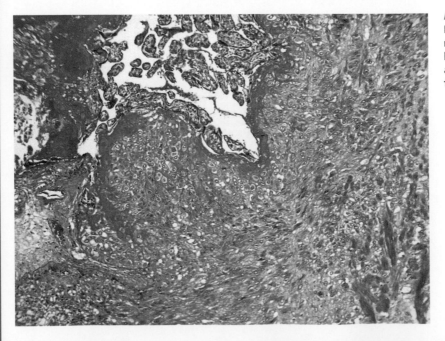

Fig. 11. Placenta accreta—Nitabuch fibrin and intermediate trophoblast are between placental tissue and myometrium (hematoxylin-eosin).

Fig. 12. Smooth muscle actin stains the muscle fibers adherent to the basal plate in this case of accreta (antibody to smooth muscle actin).

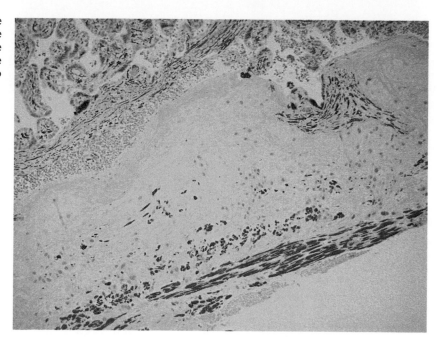

trophoblast at the implantation site from basal decidua (**Table 2**),[36] also complicating the issue. Decidual cells are individually surrounded by reticulin, whereas intermediate trophoblast does not form a reticulin network but disrupts the reticulin of the myometrium (**Figs. 17** and **18**).[36]

Extravillous trophoblast may also be distinguished by keratin positivity in trophoblast but not decidua (**Fig. 19**).[8] It often takes many sections to establish a diagnosis. Villi in direct contact with myometrium are helpful but not a requisite of diagnosis, because much fibrinoid

Fig. 13. Placenta increta showing placental tissue extending into myometrium (hematoxylin-eosin).

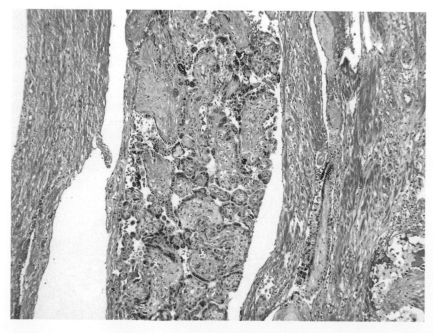

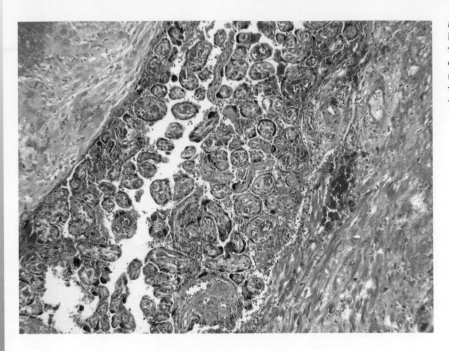

Fig. 14. Placenta increta—it is unusual to be able to obtain sections of placenta surrounded by rather than thinning out the myometrium (hematoxylin-eosin).

and extravillous trophoblast may be seen in continuity with villi. The hallmark of histologic diagnosis is absence of decidua, and if the villi are admixed with extravillous trophoblast and fibrinoid, which is then in contact with myometrium without any decidua present, the diagnosis is made.[8] Presence of extravillous trophoblast and placental site giant cells (multinucleated intermediate trophoblast) in myometrium is not an indication of accreta. The decidual layer away from a focal or partial accreta is generally unremarkable.

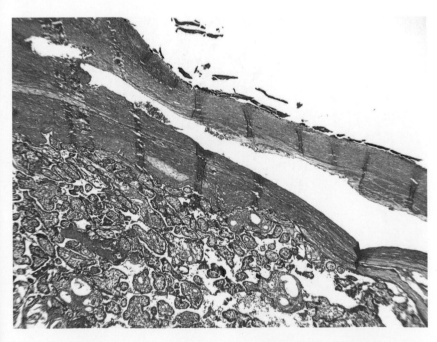

Fig. 15. Placenta percreta—a thin rim of residual myometrium is seen in this section adjacent to the area of total placental penetration of the uterine wall (hematoxylin-eosin).

Fig. 16. Placenta percreta. Ink was applied to the outside uterine surface. Often sections come out disrupted, such as this one. Placental tissue is seen at the ink (hematoxylin-eosin).

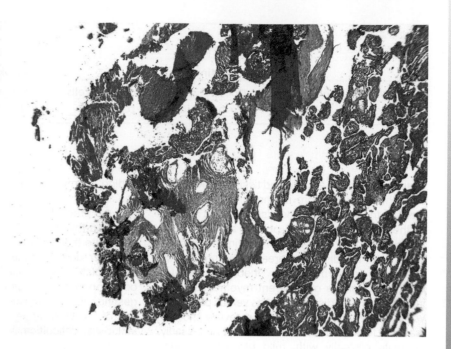

Placenta increta is the invasion of the placental tissue into the myometrium. In distinction from invasive mole, the villi are normal (**Table 3**). Placenta percreta is the full-thickness penetration of the placental tissue. These diagnoses are often easier to make grossly than histologically. As the placenta invades beyond the surface of the uterine cavity, the myometrium is more likely to appear thinned out, rather than invaded, resulting in histologic sections that rarely show villi surrounded by muscle. With placenta percreta, applying ink to the uterine serosa may provide a section where the placental tissue is seen at the ink. If a few strands of muscle remain, muscle stains may highlight them.

Stanek[42] has postulated that there is a missing link lesion, occult placenta accreta, where asymptomatic patients have myometrial fibers attached to spontaneously delivered placentas, basing the theory on increased numbers of intermediate trophoblasts in these placentas compared with controls stained with CD146. Jacques and colleagues[43] described a series of similar cases they considered milder forms of accreta, diagnosed by myometrium on the basal plate of the placenta, with decidual deficiency. They reported that a diagnosis of accreta was only occasionally clinically suspected, but clinical risk factors were similar to clinically apparent cases, and more than half of the patients in their series required manual removal of the placenta. Complications included retained placenta and postpartum hemorrhage, but none of the patients went on to hysterectomy. Khong and Werger[41] postulated that grossly disrupted placental areas correlate

Table 1
Differential diagnosis of placenta accreta and exaggerated placental site

Diagnosis	Common Features	Distinguishing Features
Accreta	Exuberant IT in decidua and myometrium	Villi in contact with myometrium or admixed with IT and fibrinoid in presence of deficient decidua
Exaggerated placental site	Exuberant IT in decidua and myometrium	Villi if present are separated from myometrium by decidua

Table 2
Distinction of intermediate trophoblast and decidua

	Reticulin	Cytokeratin	Vimentin
Intermediate trophoblast	Does not surround individual cells	Positive	Negative
Decidua	Surrounds individual cells	Negative	Positive

to areas of accreta and studied tissue blocks taken from these areas, from normal areas, and from areas at the interface of the disrupted and normal. In their study, the mixed normal and disrupted areas yielded the most likely site to find myometrial fibers, with the disrupted areas alone not fruitful. They also confirmed their theory of greater numbers of cases of adherent myometrial fibers in placentas with disrupted areas versus placentas without such areas. Clinical chart review showed that this finding can confirm, but not necessarily correlate clinically with, mild placenta accreta. Their finding of myometrial fibers in approximately 30% of placentas, probably correlated with their extensive research sectioning protocol, performed prospectively. They found high rates of myometrial fibers in en face (shaved) blocks of the basal plate, which sampled significantly larger areas of basal plate than conventional sections, but noted the risk of losing the area in question with trimming of a block. Their final conclusion was that the

finding of myometrial fibers on the basal plate can confirm a clinical impression of accreta or may be present in the absence of clinical suspicion, but the absence of such muscle fibers does not refute the clinical diagnosis.

Sherer and colleagues[44] noted that placental basal plate myometrial fibers were 10 times as common in preterm births as in term births, suggesting this may explain the increased abnormalities of the third stage of labor in preterm births, including difficulties with placental separation and increased bleeding, and may somehow relate to accreta but noted that myometrial fibers seen at the basal plate did not definitively diagnose accreta. There is a higher association of retained placenta after second trimester deliveries.[45]

It has been recommended that these milder and potentially clinically unapparent cases of accreta diagnosed by the presence of myometrial fibers on the basal plate be acknowledged in the pathology report, because they may serve as

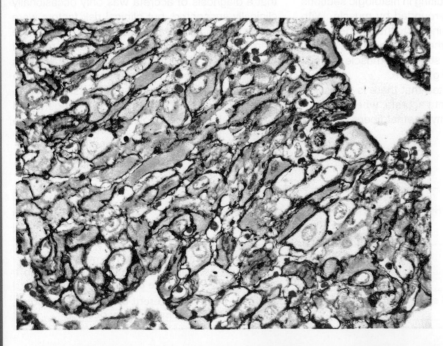

Fig. 17. Reticulin stain outlines individual decidual cells (reticulin stain).

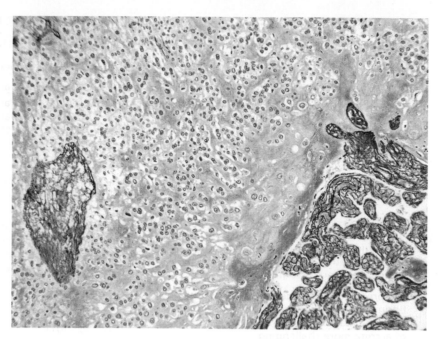

Fig. 18. Reticulin stain does not outline the intermediate trophoblast (reticulin stain).

a warning of postpartum complications or risk of creta in a subsequent pregnancy.[46]

Additional histologic findings in accreta may include focal deficiency of physiologic conversion of spiral arterioles and deficient placental septum formation, which, if present, may be composed of myometrium rather than extravillous trophoblast, fibrinoid, and decidua.[8]

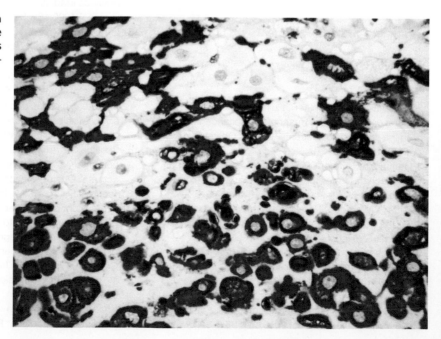

Fig. 19. Keratin stain delineates intermediate trophoblast but does not stain decidua (Antibody to cytokeratin).

Table 3
Differential diagnosis of placenta increta/percreta and invasive hydatidiform mole

Diagnosis	Common Features	Distinguishing Features
Placenta increta/percreta	Villi within myometrium	Villi are normal
Invasive mole	Villi within myometrium	Villi are molar, with hydropic change and trophoblast proliferation

Pitfalls
IN THE DIAGNOSIS OF
PLACENTA ACCRETA/PERCRETA

! Lack of identification of villi in direct contact with myometrium does not rule out accreta. Decidual absence is confirmatory.

! The presence of intermediate trophoblast and fibrinoid between placental tissue and myometrium may make the histologic diagnosis of accreta more challenging.

! Extravillous trophoblast should not be interpreted as decidua.

! Presence of extravillous trophoblasts and placental site giant cells in the myometrium should not be overinterpreted as evidence of accreta/increta.

! Myometrium may be thinned out rather than histologically invaded in increta/percreta.

! Careless handling of a hysterectomy specimen may disrupt the site of placenta percreta.

REFERENCES

1. Khong TY. The pathology of placenta accreta, a worldwide epidemic. J Clin Pathol 2008;61: 1243–6.
2. Warshak CR, Eskander R, Hull AD, et al. Accuracy of ultrasonography and magnetic resonance imaging in the diagnosis of placenta accreta. Obstet Gynecol 2006;108:573–81.
3. Tantbirojn P, Crum CP, Parast MM. Pathophysiology of placenta creta: the role of decidua and extravillous trophoblast. Placenta 2008;29:639–45.
4. Titiz H, Wallace A, Voaklander DC. Manual removal of the placenta—a case control study. Aust N Z J Obstet Gynaecol 2001;41:41–4.
5. Blanchette H. The rising cesarean delivery rate in America. What are the consequences. Obstet Gynecol 2011;118:687–90.
6. Silver RM, Landon MB, Rouse DT, et al. Maternal morbidity associated with multiple repeat cesarean delivery. Obstet Gynecol 2006;107:1226–32.

7. Al-Khan A, Aye IL, Barsoum A, et al. IFPA meeting 2010 workshops report II: placental pathology;trophoblast invasion, fetal sex; parasites and the placenta; decidua and embryonic or fetal loss; trophoblast differentiation and syncytialization. Placenta 2011;32(Suppl 2):s90–9.
8. Baergen RN. Postpartum Hemorrhage, subinvolution of the placental site, and placenta accreta. In: Baergen RN, editor. Manual of pathology of the human placenta. 2nd edition. New York: Springer; 2011. p. 192–9.
9. Esh-Broder E, Ariel I, Abas-Bashir N, et al. Placenta accreta is associated with IVF pregnancies: a retrospective chart review. BJOG 2011;118:1084–9.
10. Thiel DH, Grodin JM, Ross GT, et al. Partial placenta accreta in pregnancies following chemotherapy for gestational trophoblastic neoplasms. Am J Obstet Gynecol 1972;112:54–8.
11. Morken NH, Henriksen H. Placenta percreta-two cases and review of the literature. Eur J Obstet Gynecol Reprod Biol 2001;100:112–5.
12. Pridjian G, Rich NE, Montag AG. Pregnancy haemoperitoneum and placenta percreta in a patient with previous irradiation and ovarian failure. Am J Obstet Gynecol 1990;162:1205–6.
13. El-Miligy M, Gordon A, Houston G. Focal myometrial defect and partial placenta accreta in a pregnancy following bilateral uterine artery embolization. J Vasc Interv Radiol 2007;18:789–91.
14. Eller AG, Bennett MA, Sharshiner M, et al. Maternal morbidity in cases of placenta accreta managed by a multidisciplinary care team compared with standard obstetric care. Obstet Gynecol 2011;117:331–7.
15. Sentilhes L, Ambroselli C, Kayem G, et al. Maternal outcome after conservative treatment of placenta accreta. Obstet Gynecol 2010;115:526–34.
16. Tseng JJ, Chou MM, Hsieh YT, et al. Differential expression of vascular endothelial growth factor, placenta growth factor and their receptors in placentae from pregnancies complicated by placenta accreta. Placenta 2006;27:70–8.
17. Cohen M, Wuillemin C, Irion O, et al. Role of decidua in trophoblastic invasion. Neuro Endocrinol Lett 2010;31:193–7.
18. Khong TY, Robertson WB. Placenta creta and placenta praevia creta. Placenta 1987;8:399–409.

19. Garmi G, Goldman S, Shalev E, et al. The effects of decidual injury on the invasion potential of trophoblastic cells. Obstet Gynecol 2011;1:55–9.

20. Earl U, Bulmer JN, Briones A. Placenta accreta: an immunohistological study of trophoblast populations. Placenta 1987;8:273–82.

21. Kim KR, Jun SY, Kim JY, et al. Implantation site intermediate trophoblasts in placenta cretas. Mod Pathol 2004;17:1483–90.

22. Li H, Cheung AN, Tsao SW, et al. Expression of e-cadherin and beta-catenin in trophoblastic tissue in normal and pathological pregnancies. Int J Gynecol Pathol 2003;22:63–70.

23. Beuker JM, Erwich JJ, Khong TY. Is endomyometrial injury during termination of pregnancy or curettage following miscarriage the precursor to placenta accreta? J Clin Pathol 2005;58:273–5.

24. Gielchinsky Y, Rojansky N, Fasouliotis SJ, et al. Placenta accreta—summary of 10 years: a survey of 310 cases. Placenta 2002;23:210–4.

25. Papadakis JC, Christodoulou N. Placenta percreta presenting in the first trimester: review of the literature. Clin Exp Obstet Gynecol 2008;35:98–102.

26. Rashbaum WK, Gates EJ, Jones J, et al. Placenta accreta encountered during dilatation and evacuation in the second trimester. Obstet Gynecol 1995;85:701–3.

27. Gherman RB, McBrayer S, Tichnor J, et al. Placenta increta complication first-trimester D&C. Obstet Gynecol 1999;93:845.

28. Oyelese Y, Smulian JC. Placenta previa, placenta accreta, and vasa previa. Obstet Gynecol 2006;107:927–41.

29. Washecka R, Behling A. Urologic complications of placenta percreta invading the urinary bladder: a case report and review of the literature. Hawaii Med J 2002;61:66–9.

30. Walter AJ, McCullough AE, Patel MD, et al. Placenta increta presenting as delayed postabortal hemorrhage. Obstet Gynecol 1999;93:846.

31. Warshak CR, Ramos GA, Eskander R, et al. Effect of predelivery diagnosis in 99 consecutive cases of placenta accreta. Obstet Gynecol 2010;115:65–9.

32. Hung T, Shau W, Hsieh C, et al. Risk factors for placenta accreta. Obstet Gynecol 1999;93:545–50.

33. Kupfermink MJ, Tamura RK, Wigton TR, et al. Placenta accreta is associated with elevated maternal serum alpha-fetoprotein. Obstet Gynecol 1993;82:266–9.

34. Comstock CH. Antenatal diagnosis of placenta accreta: a review. Ultrasound Obstet Gynecol 2005;26:89–96.

35. Kim H, Hill MC, Winick AB, et al. Prenatal diagnosis of placenta accreta with pathologic correlation. Radiographics 1998;18:237–42.

36. Morison JE. Placenta Accreta: a clinicopathologic review of 67 cases. Obstet Gynecol Annu 1978;7:107–23.

37. Davis JD, Cruz A. Persistent placenta increta: a complication of conservative management of presumed placenta accreta. Obstet Gynecol 1996;88:653–4.

38. Pacheco LD, Gei AF. Controversies in the management of placenta accreta. Obstet Gynecol Clin North Am 2011;38:313–22.

39. Mazouni C, Gorincour G, Juhan V, et al. Placenta accreta: a review of current advances in prenatal diagnosis. Placenta 2007;28:599–603.

40. El Behery MM, Rasha LE, El Alfy Y. Cell-free placental mRNA in maternal plasma to predict placental invasion in patients with placenta accreta. Int J Gynaecol Obstet 2010;109:30–3.

41. Khong TY, Werger AC. Myometrial fibers in the placental basal plate can confirm but do not necessarily indicate clinical placenta accreta. Am J Clin Pathol 2001;116:703–8.

42. Stanek J. Occult placenta accreta: the missing link in the diagnosis of abnormal placentation. Pediatr Dev Pathol 2007;10:266–73.

43. Jacques SM, Qureshi F, Trent VS, et al. Placenta accreta: mild cases diagnosed by placental examination. Int J Gynecol Pathol 1996;15:28–33.

44. Sherer DM, Salafia CM, Minior VK, et al. Placental basal plate myometrial fibers: clinical correlations of abnormally deep trophoblast invasion. Obstet Gynecol 1996;87:444–9.

45. Sunaram S, Diaz JP, Gonzalez-Quintero VH, et al. Rectal misoprostol vs 15-methyl prostaglandin F2 alpha for retained placenta after second-trimester delivery. Am J Obstet Gynecol 2009;200:e24–6.

46. Faye-Petersen OM, Heller DS, Joshi VV. Lesions of the placenta as a whole. In: Faye-Petersen OM, Heller DS, Joshi VV, editors. Handbook of placental pathology. 2nd edition. Abingdon, Oxon (United Kingdom): Taylor & Francis; 2006. p. 88.

Index

Note: Page numbers of article titles are in **boldface** type.

A

Abruption, chronic, 165–166
    pathologic characteristics of, 164–165
    risk for cerebral palsy, 164
    subacute and/or chronic, 163
Abruptio placenta/uterine rupture, birth asphyxia and
    neonatal encephalopathy and, 154–156
    sentinel events in, 158
Acute chorioamnionitis (ACA), fetal inflammatory
    response in, 38–41, 43–44
        at chorionic plate vessels, 39
        differential diagnosis of, 46–52
        early, 39–40, 42
        in necrotizing funisitis, 40–41, 43
        mild to moderate, chorionic vasculitis in, 41,
          43–44
        neutrophil infiltration of umbilical arteries, 39,
          42
        severe, funisitis in, 40–41, 43
        umbilical vein *vs.* umbilical vasculitis with
          arterial involvement, 39–40, 42
        vs. eosinophilic/T-cell chorionic vasculitis,
          46–48
        vs. meconium-associated vascular necrosis
          with inflammation, 48–49
        vs. umbilical pseudovasculitis, 51–52
        vs. villitis of unknown etiology with obliterative
          fetal vasculopathy, 47, 49–50
    gross features of, 35
        appearance of fetal placental surface, 36
        necrotizing funisitis, 36
    identification of infectious organisms in, 43, 45
    infectious organisms in, 43, 45
        Fusobacterium sp., 45
    key points for pathology report, 37
    maternal inflammatory response in, 37–39
        differential diagnosis of, 45–46
        grading of, 40–41
        in initial phase, neutrophils and trophoblast
          layer, 37–38
        microabscesses in, 37, 41
        polymorphonuclear leukocytes in, 38
        severe, 37, 40
        vs. chronic chorioamnionitis, 45–46
        vs. laminar necrosis, 45
        vs. necrotizing chorioamnionitis, 37, 39
    microscopic features of, 35–37
    overview of, frequency of, 33–34
        key diagnostic criteria for, 33–34
        pathogenesis of, 34
        placental inflammation from, 34–35
        risk factors for, 34
        spontaneous preterm birth and, 35
    pitfalls/differential diagnosis of, 175–176
    placental inflammation patterns in, 51–57

B

Beckwith-Wiedmann syndrome, placentas in, 32,
    147–148

C

Chorionamnionitis, acute, **33–60** (*See Acute
    chorioamnionitis*)
    chronic, 45–46
Chronic histiocytic intervillositis. *See Massive chronic
    intervillositis (MCI).*

D

Distal villous immaturity (DVI), 168–169
    relation to CNS injury, 168
    with multifocal chorangiomatosis, 168

E

Eosinophilic/T-cell chorionic vasculitis, frequency of, 47
    microscopic appearance of, 47–48
    villitis of unknown etiology in, 47
    vs. acute chorioamnionitis, 46–49
Erythroblastic response to reduced fetal oxygen
    tension, 175

F

Fetal hemorrhage, fetomaternal hemorrhage,
    155–156
    from lacerations, 156–157
    intervillous thrombi/hemorrhages, 157
    stem villous arteriolar constriction and venular
        dilatation, 157–158
Fetal inflammatory response, to amniotic bacterial
    infection, neurologic impairments, 172
        nonocclusive chorionic vessel thrombosis,
          172–173
        perinatal stroke, 172–173
        severe acute chorionic vasculitis, 173
        umbilical arteritis, 172

Surgical Pathology 6 (2013) 199–203
http://dx.doi.org/10.1016/S1875-9181(13)00009-3
1875-9181/13/$ – see front matter © 2013 Elsevier Inc. All rights reserved.

Fetal meconium release, meconium-associated
  vascular necrosis from, 174–175
  prolonged, 173–174
  recent, 173–174
Fetal thrombotic vasculopathy (FTV), **87–100,**
  159–160, 162
  clinical features of, 88
    risk factors for, 88–89
  differential diagnosis of, summary of, 97
    vs. chronic villitis with obliterative fetal
      vasculopathy, 94–95
    vs. infarct, 96–97
    vs. intrauterine fetal death, 94
    vs. mesenchymal dysplasia, 95–96
  gross features of, chorionic plate vessels, 88–89
    morphologic, 89
    obstructive lesions of cord, 88
    pale triangular regions in, 88–89
  impact on outcome
    growth restriction, 98
    hypoxic-ischemic encephalopathy, 97
    in neonatal stroke, 97
  impact on outcome, esophageal atresia, 97–98
  key features of, 87
  microscopic features of, blood cell extravasation
    with fibrin accumulation, 90–91
    calcification in vessel wall and in clot, 90, 92
    chronic villous changes, 93
    fibrinous vasculosis, 90
    hemorrhagic endovasculopathy, 91, 92–93
    intimal fibrin cushions, 90–91
    iron deposition in basement membrane, 93–94
    layered blood elements in, 990
    red cell extravasation into villous stroma,
      93–94
    septation pattern, 90–91
  prevalence of, 87–88
Fetal vasculopathy(ies), fetal thrombotic, 159–160
  early stage, 160
  relation to CNS injury, 160
  villitis of unknown etiology with obliterative fetal
    vasculopathy, 159–161
  meconium-associated vascular necrosis with
    inflammation, histopathologic features of,
    48–49
  umbilical or chorionic fetal large vessel, 48

M

Massive chronic intervillositis (MCI), **115–126**
  clinical outcomes of, 124
  diagnosis of, association with villitis of unknown
    origin, 124
  differential diagnosis of, infectious cuases in,
    123–124
  etiology of, 124
  histologic characterization of, 123

key features of, 123
Massive perivillous fibrin deposition (MPVFD)
  diagnosis of, gross features in, 106–107
    patterns in placental pathology report in, 107
  differential diagnosis of, 110
    vs. avascular villi and chronic villitis, 107–109–7
    vs. chorionic villous ischemia and infarction,
      107–108
    vs. diffuse villitis of unknown etiology, 107–109
    vs. massive chorionic intervillositis, 107–109
    vs. perivillous fibrinoid deposition, 107
  gross features of, after fixation, 102–104
    in classic maternal floor infarction, 103
    maternal surface in, 101–102
    parenchyma of, 102–104
    yellowish basal layer or rind of fibrinoid in,
      101–103
  impact of, 111
  key points in, 102
  microscopic features of, basal surface and
    placental parenchyma, 103, 105
    extravillous cytotrophoblast and X-cell
      proliferations in, 103, 105–106
    progression of, 105
    scattered lymphocytes and monocyte/
      histiocytes, 105–106
  pathogenesis of, 111–112
    maternal autoimmune or alloimmune condition,
      111
    maternal inherited coagulation factor
      deficiencies in, 111
  pitfalls in, 112
Maternal floor infarction (MFI), **101–114.** *See Massive
  perivillous fibrin deposition (MPVFD).*
Maternal malperfusion (MMP), definition/
  pathogenesis of, 166
  pathological characteristics of, distal villous
    hypoplasia/undergrowth, 167–168
    villous infarcts, 166–167
  risk for cerebral palsy and neuroencephalopathy,
    166
Meconium-associated vascular necrosis (MAVN),
  174–175
  pitfalls/differential diagnosis of, 175–176
Monoxygotic twinning, acardiac twins and, 30–31
  and Beckwith-Wiedmann syndrome, 31–32
  conjoined twins and, 31
  development of, 27–28
  key features of, 28
  monoamniotic, 28–29
  monoamniotic *vs.* dichorionic, 29
  twin-to-twin transfusion syndrome in, 29
    gross pathology of, 30
    irregular splitting of embryolasts i30n
    laser ablation therapy in, 29–30
  vanishing twins and, 31
Monozygotic twinning, **27–32**

P

Partial asphyxia/chronic intermittent hypoxia,
162–163
abruption, subacute/chronic, 165–166
from chronic partial/intermittent umbilical cord
compression, 163–164
Perivillous fibrin(oid) deposition, neurodevelopmental
abnormalities from, 169–170
rapidly evolving pattern in, 170
slowly evolving pattern in, 171
vs. perivillous plaques, 171
Placenta, correlation of pathology with perinatal brain
injury, **153–180**
fetal surface vessels of, thrombosis of, 16–17
gross examination of, **1–26**
formalin fixation for, 1–2
steps in, 26
systematic procedure for, 1–2
gross lesions of, fetal surface, 9, 11
peripheral membranes, 9–11
placental weight and, 3
placenta previa, 3–4
umbilical cord in, 4–10
mesenchymal dysplasia of, **127–151**
villous tissue and maternal surface of, avascular
villi, 23–25
blood clots on, 19, 21
calcification, 16, 18
central and large infarcts, 16, 19
chorangiomas, 24–25
cystic change in infarcts, 16
hydrops fetalis, 16, 18
intervillous thrombi, 23
large central and marginal infarcts, 16–20
perivillous firin deposition, 23–24
retroplacental hemorrhage, 19–22
villous infarcts, 16, 19
Placenta accreta/percreta, **181–197**
accreta, differential diagnosis of, 189, 193
distinction of intermediate trophoblast and
decidua in, 191, 194–195
etiology of, 182–183
microscopic diagnosis of, 187, 189–191
therapy for, conservative vs. hysterectomy,
185
clinical diagnosis of, bladder involvement in, 184
intrapartum hemorrhage, 183–184
defined, 181
differential diagnosis of placenta increta/percreta
and invasive hydatidiform mole, 196
increta, microscopic diagnosis of, 187–188,
191–193
MRI findings in, 184–185
pathologic diagnosis of, gross appearance in,
186–188
microscopic, 187–196

percreta, microscopic diagnosis of, 188, 192–193
pitfalls in diagnosis of, 196
rising incidence of, 181
treatment of, 182
ultrasound findings in, 184–185
Placental biomarker lesions, acute chorioamnionitis,
176
meconium-related changes, 176
Placental mesenchymal dysplasia, characteizaton
of, 127–128
clinical correlations and clinicopathogenetic
implications of, Beckwith-Wiedemann
syndrome, 147–148
infant mesenchymal harmatomas, 148
intrauterine growth restriction, 147–148
diagnosis of, 128, 145–147
androgenetic-biparental mosaicism in,
145–148
histopathologic findings in, 144
p57kip immunohistochemistry in, 146–147
differential diagnosis of, 138–145
vs. chorangiomas, chorangiomatosis,
135–137, 140
vs. complete hydatidiform mole, 141, 143
vs. fetaoplacental hydrops, 142–145
vs. multifocal chorangiomatosis, 136–137, 140
vs. partial hydatidform mole, 140–141
vs. subchorionic cysts, 140–141
vs. subchorionic cysts/thrombohematomas,
141–142, 144
gross features of, 128–130
Beckwith-Wiedemann syndrome-associated,
130
cystic villi in, 130–133
suggestive of partial mole, 130
histopathology of, 132–133
key points, 127
microscopic features of, anomalous stem villi in,
132, 136
chorangioma in, 135–137
chorangiomatosis in, 136–137
chorangiosis in, 135–137
chorionic villi in, 134, 137
cistern formations in, 132, 136
complicated by fetal vasculopathy, 134, 137
erythroblastosis in, 137–138
fetal nucleated red blood cells in, 137–138
fetal thrombotic vasulopathic lesions in, 134, 137
fetomaternal hemorrhage in, 138, 140
fibromatous villi in, 134, 136
histopathology of, 132–133
with fibromatous villous stroma, 134, 136
Placental pathology correlated with perinatal brain
injury, gross description of, histologic evaluation
in, 154
synoptic elements in, 154

Placental (*continued*)
  lgorithm for relating placental findings to
      neurologic outcome, 178
  overview of, placental processes in, 153–154
  placental biomarkers and, erythroblastic response
      to reduced fetal oxygen tension, 175–176
    fetal inflammatory response to bacterial
        infection, 172–173
  placental syndromes, abruption, subacute and/or
      chronic, 163–165
    chronic villitis with obliterative fetal
        vasculopathy, 159–162
    distal villous immaturity, 168–169
    fetal thrombotic vasculopathy, 159–160
    fetal vasculopathies, key features of, 162
    maternal malperfusion, 166–168
    perivillous fibrin(oid) deposition, 169–171
    pitfalls/differential diagnosis of, 162–163, 165,
        170–171
    prolonged partial asphyxia/chronic intermittent
        hypoxia, 162–163
    umbilical cord compression, chronic partial/
        intermittent, 163–164
    uteroplacental insufficiency/decreased
        placental reserve, 165–171
  placental syndromes with fetal vasculopathies,
      158
    genomic storms in, 158
  sentinel events/total asphyxia, abruptio placenta/
      uterine rupture, 154–155
    birth asphyxia and, 154
    categories of, 154
    complete umbilical cord occlusion, 155–156
    fetal hemorrhage, 155–157
    fetomaternal hemorrhage, 155–156
    intervillous thrombi/hemorrhages, 157–158
    key features of, 158
    lacerations, 156–157
    pitfalls/differetial diagnosis of, 158
  synthesis of placental findings and neurologic
      outcome, 177–178
  timing of, 177

U

Umbilical cord, **61–85**
  aneurysms or varices in, 77
  coiling of, evaluation of degree, 62, 67–68
  constriction of, 67–68
  discoloration of, brown in hemosiderin deposition,
      63
    green in prebirth meconium discharge, 62–63
    in acute funisitis, 63, 65
    in candidal infection, 63, 66
    red from hemolysis, 63–64
    yellow in maternal bilirubinemia, 63–64
  embryonic remnants of, allantoic duct, 78–80

allantoic duct cyst in, 79–80
    of other tissues, 80–81
    omphalomesenteric or vitelline duct, 79–81
  entanglement of, 70–71
    fetal demise from, 70
  fetal amnion surface, amnion nodosum at,
      11, 14
    oligohydramnios with denuded chorionic plate
        on, 11, 13
    squamous metaplasia on, 11, 14
  fetal placental amnion membrane in, 9
  fetal surface, cysts on, 11–12
    fibrin deposits from maternal circulation on, 11
  fetal surface amnion membrane, color and
      translucency of, 14–15
  hemangiomas and other neoplasms in, histologic
      appearance of, 82
    sequealae of, 82–83
  hematoma in, causes of, 77
    consequences of, 77
    gross appearance of, 77
  insertion of, 62
    furcate, 71–72
    interpositional, 71–72
    velamentous, 71–73
      hemorrhage from, 71, 73
      vasa previa and, 73
  knots in, false, 68–69
    true, 62, 68–69
  length of, determination of, 64–65
    excessive, 65, 67
    functionally short, 64–65
    long, 63
    short, 65
  lesions in, absence of an artery in, 4
    chronic necrotizing funisitis, 7, 9
    division into branch vessels, 7, 9
    edema of, 5–6
    hemorrhage in, 9
    left twist of, 4–5
    long cord, 5–6
    microabscesses in *Candida* infection, 7, 9
    short cord, 5
    staining with meconium exposure, 7, 10
    structure of, 5, 7
    thrombosis of artery with barberpole
        appearance, 7, 9–10
    velamentous insertion with compression or
        rupture, 5, 7
  meconium-associated myonecrosis of, 81–82
  membrane discoloration, from exposed placenta,
      14
    from mecomium passage, 14–15
    from old hemorrhage, 15–17
  microscopic lesions and features of, 78–83
  peripheral chorion in, 9–10
    subchorionic cyst in, 12

peripheral margin of, circummargination, 11
   circumvallation in, 11, 13
prolapse of, 71
remnant of yolk sac between amnion and chorion
   in, 10–11
rupture of, 77–78
single umbilical artery in, 62, 73–74
   cross sections of, 74
   microscopic section of, 74
   supernumerary, 72, 75
thrombi in, 99
thrombosis of umbilical vessels in, 76–77
   gross identification of, 76
   microscopic, 76–77
Umbilical cord occlusion, occlusion of fetal vascular
   blood flow to head in, 155–156
   retained flow in umbilical arteries, 155, 157
Umbilical cord pathology, description of, 61
   gross examination and pathology of, 61–62
   gross lesions and features in, coiling, 65,
      67–68
      cord discoloration, 62–63
      cord length, 63–67
      entanglement, 70–71
      hematoma, 76–77
      hemorrhage, differential diagnosis of, 76
      insertion, 71–73
      knots, 68–69
      prolapse, 71
      rupture, 77–78
      single artery, 73–74
      structure, 65, 67–68
      supernumerary vessels, 75
      thrombosis of umbilical arteries, 75–77
   microscopic, key points in, 77
   microscopic lesions and features, embryonic
      remnants, 78–81

hemangiomas, 82–83
meconium-associated myonecrosis, 81–82
teratomas, 83
Uteroplacental insufficiency/decreased placental
   reserve, 165–166
   and CNS injury, 165–166
   distal villous immaturity, 168–169
   maternal malperfusion, 166–167, 166–168

V

Villitis of unknown etiology (VUE), 115–123, **115–126**.
   See also Massive chronic intervillositis (MCI).
   characterization of, 115–119
      avascular villi in, 116, 118
      giant cells in histiocytic infiltrate, 116–117
      lymphocytic infiltrate in, 116–117
      lymphohistiocytic infiltrate in, 116
      mononuclear infiltrate in, 116
      pattern in, 116, 118
      villitis of anchoring villi in, 116, 119
      villous stromal karyorrhexis in, 116, 118
   clinical outcomes with, intrauterine growth
      restriction, 122–123
   diagnosis of, pitfalls in, 122
      sampling of placenta for, 119–120
      spectrum in, 120–121
   etiology of, graft-*versus*-host hypothesis for, 122
      unidentified infection, 122
   vs. infectious villitis, 117–118, 121
      cytomegalovirus, 118, 120
      histiologic features in, 119
      parvovirus, 118, 120
      Toxoplasma cysts, 118, 121
Villitis of unkown etiology (VUE) with obliterative fetal
   vasculopathy (OFV), 159–161
   cerebral palsy and neuroencephalopathy from, 159

Moving?

Make sure your subscription moves with you!

To notify us of your new address, find your **Clinics Account Number** (located on your mailing label above your name), and contact customer service at:

Email: journalscustomerservice-usa@elsevier.com

800-654-2452 (subscribers in the U.S. & Canada)
314-447-8871 (subscribers outside of the U.S. & Canada)

Fax number: 314-447-8029

Elsevier Health Sciences Division
Subscription Customer Service
3251 Riverport Lane
Maryland Heights, MO 63043

*To ensure uninterrupted delivery of your subscription, please notify us at least 4 weeks in advance of move.

Printed and bound by CPI Group (UK) Ltd, Croydon, CR0 4YY

03/10/2024

01040347-0001